Vital Sensation Manual

UNIT ONE:
CASETAKING

Based on
The Sensation Method
& Classical Homeopathy

Written
by
Melissa Burch, CCH & Susana Aikin, CCH

Edited by Ingrid Dankmeyer, Didi Pershouse and Sharon Willis

Cover Design by Chetana Deorah

Text Design by Janet Innes and George Papargyris

Published by
Inner Health, Inc.
175 Harvey St., #13
Cambridge, MA 02140
(617) 491-3374
melissa@innerhealth.us
www.innerhealth.us

TABLE OF CONTENTS

A. THE OLD METHOD VS. THE NEW METHOD

In this search for a homoeopathic specific remedy, that is to say, in this comparison of the collective symptoms of the natural disease with the list of symptoms of known medicines, in order to find among these an artificial morbific agent corresponding by similarity to the disease to be cured, the more striking, singular, uncommon and peculiar (characteristic) signs and symptoms of the case of disease are chiefly and most solely to be kept in view; for it is more particularly these that very similar ones in the list of symptoms of the selected medicine must correspond to, in order to constitute it the most suitable for effecting the cure. The more general and undefined symptoms: loss of appetite, headache, debility, restless sleep, discomfort, and so forth, demand but little attention when of that vague and indefinite character, if they cannot be more accurately described, as symptoms of such a general nature are observed in almost every disease and from almost every drug.

Samuel Hahnemann
§153, Organon of Medicine
Translated by R. E. Dudgeon

Traditionally since Hahnemann, homeopaths have sought to find the strange, rare and peculiar in a case as a way to find an accurate prescription for the patient. In this sense casetaking has always been directed toward exploring the minute details of a case in order to find an essential element that would lead to the remedy. Keynotes of remedies were one attempt to describe quintessential features of potentized substances. In the last couple of decades, homeopaths have used mental and emotional characteristics to recognize the patient's total state and to ultimately differentiate remedies. Even more recently, a deeper understanding of the mental and emotional state led to defining the core delusion of cases as one method of reaching an accurate prescription. It was at this point that homeopaths delved into the sections of Mind and Dreams of the repertory as probably never before, and found great remedies for many of their cases.

In the past, the homeopath would let the patient describe his problems, physical or emotional, while he would be picking up peculiar symptoms and striving to get to the bottom of the mental state. The emphasis was mainly on understanding emotional phenomena, and then confirming the picture with physicals and generals. However, this often proved a difficult and confusing task, especially when the listener got lost in the story, rather than understanding the patient's state. The main problems of this method lay in the difficulties the homeopath may have had in avoiding any interpretation of the patient's stories or emotional states; no matter how much of an unprejudiced observer he might strive to be. When working with emotional states and delusions, determining the kingdom and miasm of a case could also be confusing in this method, and much of the "objective" case analysis ended up being subjective theory.

In order to bypass the problems of interpretation that the homeopath can face in casetaking, a new method is proposed here by which the homeopath seeks to discover a deeper level of the patient's experience, or the Vital Sensation, which leads directly to the remedy with much less possibility of interpretation or transference in the casetaking. In this new method the homeopath mainly explores the chief complaint of the patient in order to find the Vital Sensation that permeates the case at all levels.

While the former methods of casetaking tried to find the state by working from the periphery of the case to the center, the new method strives to go directly to the center and project outwards. It relies on the abstract experiential language of the patient, thus finding a way around rational and logical language, leaving very little space for conceptual elaboration; and it is therefore a more direct method and properly used will render a higher level of success in casetaking.

Why focus on the chief complaint as the main source of the Vital Sensation, instead of any other area of the patient? First of all, it is the chief complaint that drives the patient to see the homeopath; so in the mind of the patient the chief complaint is precisely what needs to be cured. Secondly, the chief complaint has always been recognized as the tip of the iceberg in a case, as the acute manifestation of the total state. If the case is looked at as a holographic paradigm, the chief complaint is a perfect holographic representation of the whole, a tiny part of the human being mirroring the totality--The microcosmic vision of the macrocosm.

By observing the chief complaint, the homeopath will be looking at an abstract picture of the totality of the state that allows for little rational, emotional or cultural interpretation. The body and the mind both express the same phenomena, the same disturbance and the same vital problem. By eliciting the raw experience or sensation of the patient in the chief complaint, the homeopath will be looking into a primal source of information, directly into the vital sphere of the case that can lead to a deeper and more accurate prescription.

This is a major shift from the earlier approach, where the homeopath would start with broad and seemingly disconnected data and then go step by step into the center. Many prescriptions were based on a collection of symptoms that would match a remedy; or sometimes a prescription would be based on discovering a common theme, like the theme of responsibility in Aurum, fear of death in Arsenicum, shock in Aconitum, etc. The concept was that themes reigned over remedies. Now the homeopath cannot talk of themes, not even of delusional states, he needs to go deeper into the case and find the quintessential energy pattern that permeates all levels of the patient's particular state, the essence that will dictate the whole prescription.

The homeopath has to find a level where language is so abstract, primal and non-human specific, that the compensation of the state does not interfere in the evaluation of the case. Here is where the Vital Sensation comes into play: something that cannot be interpreted, cannot be explained or even understood on rational grounds but expresses itself throughout the case at all levels and in all details. The Vital Sensation then becomes the master key to the whole case.

B. THE VITAL SENSATION

I used to think that the center of the mental state was the deepest point that we could reach, but with my study of plant families, I saw that the patient's delusion is not only confined to the mind but is also expressed in the physical sphere. I realized that the central state was not merely an emotion or a feeling, but a common sensation that connected the mind and the body. I call this common sensation the Vital Sensation as it is something deeper to the mind and body. In fact I could see that the mental state is merely one expression of the Vital Sensation…. I also realized that the concept of the Vital Sensation was not just confined to the plant kingdom. In the case of disease and remedy states, I perceived that this Vital Sensation exists in all the kingdoms, both at the physical and the emotional spheres.

Dr. Rajan Sankaran
An Insight into Plants

The latest development in homeopathy is to consider the chief complaint as the most direct link into the Vital Sensation of the patient, which underlies and manifests throughout all levels of the patient's state, and needs to be confirmed in every detail of the case. For example, when a person says that he feels jealous or suspicious or expresses something mental and emotional, then it is possible to ask him: What is his experience? He may feel he is being attacked and is frightened. In this way an emotional situation is perceived behind the mental symptom, which in the old method may be clear enough for a prescription. However, if the homeopath wants to take it one step further then she asks the patient how he experiences the attack. At this point the case comes to an intersection where the mind and body meet. Here the patient may have the feeling that something is breaking, burning or twisting. At this point he is describing the Vital Sensation and will express his emotional and physical symptoms in the same terms. This is a very deep level, and there is an opportunity for a much better chance of success in prescribing.

In many cases, when the patient expresses a local physical sensation in relation to the chief complaint, the same sensation emerges in the emotional sphere too. For example, the patient says, "With the knee joint pain, I feel very stiff and I cannot move," and in the emotional sphere she describes her problems with her mother-in-law in the same terms: "I feel scared (an emotion) as if she is going to attack me (a delusion). I feel extremely stiff and I just can't move." Here in the case there is "stiffness and can't move" as the Vital Sensation, which lies at a deeper level than the duality of the mind and body.

The chief complaint represents the crystallization of the Vital Sensation in the physical sphere. Hence it is the best place to locate the Vital Sensation. It is the fountainhead where all the vital phenomena are expressed in their raw form. The chief complaint cannot be neglected, because it is the main support around which the case revolves. It forms the foundation of the case.

Below the levels of Emotion and Delusion of the patient lies the level of Sensation. It is at this deeper level of Sensation that the homeopath can elicit the non-human specific language that expresses the Vital Sensation. This Vital Sensation subsequently unfolds and manifests throughout the whole case including the levels of Emotion and Delusion. In this study of the Vital Sensation, the patient's delusion is not only confined to the mind but also expressed on the physical sphere. The first hints of the Vital Sensation come through the chief complaint; and if the chief complaint is fully examined it leads back to the Vital Sensation.

The Vital Sensation can also lead the practitioner to find the kingdom in which the case lies. In the plant kingdom, the Vital Sensation is expressed in terms of sensitivity and reactivity. In the animal kingdom, the Vital Sensation is expressed through issues of survival such as victim/aggressor, competition, attractiveness, etc. In the mineral kingdom, the Vital Sensation is expressed as problems of structure, function and performance.

C. THE IMPORTANCE OF THE CHIEF COMPLAINT

In the past many homeopaths sought to understand the case by finding connecting symptoms that, when threaded together, formed the basis for a prescription. The chief complaint itself was often neglected with the belief that homeopaths should not be treating the pathology, but instead the person experiencing it. As a result of this approach, the practitioner was often impatient to get over with the chief complaint and get to the mental state of the person. Furthermore, many times homeopaths would simply get caught up in the mental phenomena without actually touching the Sensation level of the patient. In contrast, with the new approach the practitioner reaches the Vital Sensation by sticking to the chief complaint itself. Then, having unearthed the Vital Sensation at the outset of the case, it becomes clear that the whole case is just a manifold expression of this common core sensation.

The chief complaint represents a consolidation of the Vital Sensation, in the sense that it is the acute manifestation of the whole state of the patient at one given moment of space and time. It is also an abstract expression of the whole state, symbolizing the case in simplified elements that cannot be explained in rational terms or elaborated on by compensation. For example, a successful businessman has episodes of weakness (chief complaint), when he is overworked. He feels weakness (sensation) of the lower limbs. This sensation of weakness is the best place to locate the Vital Sensation. It is the fountainhead where all the vital phenomena are expressed in their raw form. It certainly cannot be neglected; it is the main support around which the case revolves. It forms the foundation of the case. The homeopath needs to stick to the chief complaint and examine it in its depth to obtain a prescription that will affect a deep cure in the case.

The chief complaint itself gives direct access to the central state of the patient, because it is a place where the homeopath can more easily lead the patient into describing sensations. These sensations, although initially appearing to only have physical connotations, can very quickly lead to discovering the Vital Sensation underlying the whole state. In many cases, when the patient expresses a local physical sensation in relation to the chief complaint, the same sensation can be seen to emerge in the emotional and mental spheres, and in the totality of the state itself.

In other cases the effect of the chief complaint on the patient's life is an expression of this Vital Sensation. For example, the patient's chief complaint is a dry cough that feels heavy and embarrasses him at work. The sensation of heaviness is expressed as a Vital Sensation and when probed the patient explains that he feels he is incapable of achieving his goals at work because he feels ashamed (level of Emotion).

In yet other cases the Vital Sensation is expressed in the modality of the chief complaint. For example, the patient has heart palpitations aggravated by any excitement, which reveals that the patient is easily affected by stimulants. In further exploration of this case, the patient has a vivid imagination, day dreams, and feels elated easily. These sensations, which initially came from the aggravation by stimulants, represent the Vital Sensation and specifically the sensations of the Rubiaceae family.

The chief complaint is often a physical complaint (arthritis, migraine, stomach ache, etc.), however, it can also present as an emotional symptom (depression, anxiety, panic attacks, etc.). This new method addresses the emotional complaint in the same manner as the physical complaint by questioning how it is experienced in the body and in the person's life, seeking to determine the Vital Sensation. For example, a patient comes with depression, and the practitioner asks how the depression is experienced in the body. The patient might respond by saying that there is a sensation of heaviness. The practitioner may also ask: How do you experience the depression in your life? And the patient might say that his life is a burden, his work load feels too heavy, and his relationships are cumbersome. At all levels the Vital Sensation relates to heaviness.

The patient's story can be very misleading in casetaking. The chief complaint, however, provides the direct experience, which points to the energy pattern and the core that underlies the case. The chief complaint represents the expression of the unbalanced vital force within the physical sphere. The sensation that emerges from the exploration of the chief complaint has to be confirmed repeatedly in the rest of the case. Therefore, the chief complaint is the central pillar of the case.

D. LAWS AND COROLLARIES

In casetaking with this new method certain laws have been noted that can help the practitioner to better understand the patient.

Three Laws

Sensation and Action are Equal and Opposite

A person's action corresponds to his perception of what is happening to him. For example, if a person feels insulted, then he would want to react by insulting. The insult could be experienced mentally or physically. If a person feels he is being injured, then he would want to injure in return, with the same intensity as he perceived the injury. He may not necessarily be aware of this or put this into action, but this will be his natural tendency.

Mercurius and *Platina* are remedies that have symptoms of homicidal impulses, and at the same time a strong fear of being killed. The desire to kill is equal and opposite to the sensation or fear that he will be killed. The remedy *Staphysagria* has the feeling of indignation and insult, and at the same time there is the symptom, *Delusion, humility and lowness of others, while he is great*.

Many remedies have symptoms of specific sensations and their corresponding actions. This law is most useful for remedies where the provings or clinical cases have not fully uncovered all the symptoms. The rubrics are partially represented in either the action or the sensation. In a remedy where only the sensation is known, the action must be equal and opposite. Sensation and action are two sides of the same coin.

The practical aspect of this law is illustrated in the following example: The patient was a woman with borderline leprosy with extensive skin lesions on both extremities. Her husband was paralyzed. She had one son, who quarreled with his wife. One day her daughter-in-law abruptly left the house after an argument and disappeared for three years. She left the patient completely alone at a time when she needed her most. Her son became depressed and stopped looking after his shop. The patient was left all alone to look after an invalid husband, a depressed son, his two small children, and the shop. When she was asked about her feelings, she said she did not feel any anger. She did not feel anything. She used to get angry and be abusive in the past but not now. Later her husband died, her daughter-in-law returned home, and her son was no longer depressed and could handle the shop. She would not express any anger for fear that her daughter-in-law might leave again. This is the time when she developed leprosy. There was such heavy suppression in her case that she developed severe pathology instead of expressing her intense emotions.

The patient had the sensation of being abandoned by her daughter-in-law, who left her completely alone when she needed her most. The main symptom is *Feels abandoned by her relatives*. In the remedy *Secale cornutum* there are the symptoms, *Delirium, abandons her relatives* and *Forsakes relations*, which is exactly the opposite of what the patient experienced. *Secale cornutum* has the symptoms represented as actions while the patient expresses the sensation. *Secale cornutum* was prescribed and the leprosy patch disappeared.

In this case the sensation is of being abandoned by her relatives and the corresponding action must be to abandon her relatives, whether she actually does it or not. Of course *Secale cornutum* has the symptom, *Forsaken feeling*, but more importantly it is the only remedy in the symptom, *Delirium, abandons her relatives*. *Forsaken feeling* explains her sensation, the single symptom explains the intensity and depth of the sensation: abandoned even by those closest to you, your own relatives. This is a common feature of remedies belonging to the Leprosy miasm, and *Secale cornutum* is one of the main remedies for treating leprosy.

In *Secale cornutum* one also finds the single symptoms, *Contemptuous, relations* for and *Mocking, relatives* his. Then it is possible to assume the opposite is true, i.e. he feels that his relatives have contempt for him and mock him, even though these sensations are not listed among the symptoms of the remedy. *Platina* is another remedy that has the symptom *Contemptuous*, which means scornful. Correspondingly it also has the symptom, *Ailments from scorn, being scorned*. So the feeling is of being scorned and the action is to be scornful.

When it is difficult to find or understand the sensation or miasm in a remedy, then it is possible to assume the sensation is equal and opposite to whatever action one finds throughout the symptomatology, and also vice versa.

The Opposite is Equally True of Whatever is Said

When a person spontaneously brings up an issue or emphasizes it, without him being asked a leading question in any direction, it means that his sensitivity is in the area of that very issue, and this sensitivity can work in two ways. If a person expresses a tremendous lack of confidence during public speaking, it means that this person is very sensitive to the issue of public speaking. On the one hand, it means that he surely lacks in confidence as he himself says, but on the other he has the potential to be a very good public speaker because of this same sensitivity to the issue. So, it is the sensitivity that makes him afraid, and it is the same sensitivity that makes him a performer. Fear and courage are, therefore, two sides of the same coin. There is proof of this example in remedies like *Argentum nitricum* or *Argentum metallicum*. People needing these remedies make the best public speakers and at the same time they can have a great fear of talking in public.

In another example, a person whose sensitivity revolves around moral issues, says that he is sensitive to cheating and doing wrong things. This most obviously means that he is affected when other people do these things, and he will not do them himself. However, it can also mean that he is capable of cheating and doing wrong things himself, the very things that he is speaking against. Sensitivity can work both ways, and so the opposite is equally true of whatever is said.

When a person emphasizes a certain issue, it means that his sensitivity lies in the area of that issue, which can only exist in relation to the opposite. For example, if an object is white it will not be visible on a white background; it can only be seen against a black background. In the same way love can exist only in the background of hate, and beauty can exist only in the background of ugliness. When a person emphasizes peace, violence must also be an issue with him. If a person talks about his positive qualities, as for example if he says that he is bold and courageous, this also means that he is fearful, and this will be expressed subconsciously, either in his dreams, hobbies, childhood etc. When a person spontaneously says that he is not afraid, it means that he is afraid. If he says that he has no fear of death, it means that he is most certainly afraid of death. Whenever someone strongly denies something, the opposite is always true. If the opposite is not true of a particular issue that issue is usually not emphasized at all.

There is No one or Nothing Out There Other Than Myself

All people function according to their individual sensitivities. Each person can perceive only what he is sensitive to, and he does not perceive at all what he is not sensitive to. So if he perceives particular qualities in others he does so because he is sensitive to these qualities. For example, if he perceives others as being contemptuous it is because his sensitivity lies in the area of contempt. People react in an equal and opposite manner to what they perceive as stated in the first law.

In the example of a person who perceives insult from another person, it is only because he is sensitive to insult that he perceives it. He cannot perceive anything other than insult. Now this person will react in an equal and opposite manner to the insult: He will react by being insulting, or at least it will be his instinct to want to insult. He sees the other person as being insulting, and he also reacts by insulting. There is no real difference between what the other person is doing and what he is doing. They are both insulting. He can see only an aspect of himself (the sensitivity to insult) in the other person and reacts only to that. This means that within him lays exactly the same person that he sees (the one who insults). Everything else lies outside of his field of perception. He sees another person as a mirror that reflects nothing but his own sensitivity, and beyond this the other person does not exist at all. So, there is no one out there but himself.

The same is true for everything around us. For example, if a person is immensely impressed by the Himalayas, the adjectives he uses to describe the mountains will have to do with his own inner sensitivity. If a person says that they are incredibly beautiful, it is very likely that his sensitivity lies in the area of beauty. He could feel he is beautiful or ugly. If, on the other hand, he says that they are immensely powerful, it is very likely that his sensitivity lies in the region of power. He could feel he is powerful or powerless. The adjectives he uses, and the meaning or the connotation they have for him, all have to do with the way he perceives himself. It could be exactly what he describes or the exact opposite.

There is hardly anything around us that is not actually a perception of our own self. If someone talks about the world coming to an end, he is basically talking about when he is going to end, because what he perceives as the end of the world is nothing but the end of himself. All of us have within us the fear of ourselves coming to an end. There was strong confirmation of this idea after seven volunteers wrote five words about the Taj

Mahal which should be as objective as possible, the way a journalist might report, in order to minimize subjectivity. Each description of the Taj Mahal was completely different from the other person's words. One person wrote that it is romantic, beautiful and sentimental. Another person described it as being grand and royal. Someone else wrote about the engineering, structures and its shape. Each person wrote and arranged the words in a way that gave an accurate picture of the person who wrote it. The different perceptions of the Taj Mahal were based on each person's perception of himself. This raises the philosophical question: Does the Taj Mahal really exist?

In the past, if the patient was strongly affected, either positively or negatively, it was important to ascertain if the patient was talking about a situation or relation that actually existed or not, then the next step would be to understand how the patient felt in that situation. What was the patient's perception of reality? Now when a patient describes a situation or other people he is only describing himself. This idea has proven very useful in practice.

Dr. Rajan Sankaran wrote in "An Insight into Plants":

> There was a family where I was treating a woman, her two daughters and also her two daughters-in-law. The daughters and daughters-in-law often visited separately and described this patient to me. Each description of the patient was so completely different that a stranger would find it difficult to believe that they were all talking about the same person. Each woman was talking about her own sensitivities and so was talking about herself rather than the patient. There was no need to ask how they felt about the patient, because their description about the woman could be repertorized and a remedy found, which proved to be a successful prescription. This case created a major change in understanding patients and their treatment.

> There was a case of a forty-year-old woman who came for treatment for ulcerative colitis. She was on heavy medication and the problem started after the death of her husband. She said her life with her husband was "pure hell." She described her husband as the most suspicious, possessive, violent and insane kind of person. He would be insanely jealous if she spoke with any other man. After obtaining an accurate description of her husband, *Hyoscyamus* was successfully prescribed. She was so affected by her husband because of her own state of jealousy and possessiveness, and her description of him reflected this sensitivity. Otherwise she would have described him in a completely different way. She saw her husband as the same remedy as she needed.

Two Corollaries:

You do to yourself what you see others do to you, and you do to others or to things what you like to do to yourself.

There is no real difference between what is seen on the outside of ourselves and what is perceived inside of us. It is only ourselves we see in others. This is true with the sensitivity to injury. In the rubric, *Striking; knocking his head against the wall*, many of the same remedies are found in the rubric, *Striking* (which means striking others). If there is a desire to injure oneself, then the person wants to do the same thing to other people or things.

Victims and aggressors are two sides of the same state. The victim has the seeds of the aggressor; and the aggressor has the victim in him.

When a person laughs at someone falling down and injuring himself in a comedy, it is because he sees himself in the injured victim. The injured victim will not provoke him to laugh unless he has a sensitivity to falling down and hurting himself. Although he is the aggressor in this case, he is also the victim. All of us have the seeds of both the aggressor and the victim within us.

A dramatic example of this corollary happened in the case of a prominent public speaker, who gave discourses on religion, and came for treatment of hypertension. Persecution was the main feeling for him, which was so strong he would become dangerously violent. When he was asked to describe the feeling of being persecuted, he said that he felt as if the people in his own house had surrounded him so that his house felt like a gas chamber. He wanted to break free but felt trapped there. He received the remedy *Drosera* which significantly improved his condition. *Drosera* has the strong feeling of being trapped and suffocated. Dorothy Shepherd suggested the same remedy for Hitler, who used the gas chamber to kill people by suffocation. This patient feels like a victim in a gas chamber, whereas Hitler was the aggressor. In general you do to your victims exactly what you feel about yourself, and conversely what you feel about yourself is what you do to others.

In this way it is possible to use sensations and their related actions in the repertories and Materia Medica interchangeably. For example, if a remedy has the rubric, *Mocking*, then the delusion of being mocked will be used even if the repertory does not list the remedy under that symptom.

Summary

Three Laws

- Sensation and action are equal and opposite.
  If a patient says some action, then be on the alert for a related sensation, or if the sensation is expressed then look for a possible action.

• The opposite is equally true of whatever is said.
  When a person emphasizes a certain issue, it means that there is sensitivity in the area of that issue. Whenever someone strongly denies something, the opposite is always true.

• There is no one or anything out there other than oneself.
  When a patient describes a situation or other people, he is only describing himself.

Two Corollaries

• You do to yourself what you see others do to you, and you do to others or to things what you like to do to yourself.

• Victims and aggressors are two sides of the same state. The victim has the seeds of aggressor, and the aggressor has the victim in him.

E. THE NEW METHOD OF CASETAKING

The approach to casetaking has changed considerably after the recent developments of the recognition of the importance of the Vital Sensation, the chief complaint and the levels of experiences. Casetaking is like a journey. It starts from the chief complaint and ends at the level of Vital Sensation. Once the practitioner has unearthed the Vital Sensation from the chief complaint, then it is possible to repeatedly find the confirmation of the Vital Sensation in all other areas of the case. The case can end at the level of Sensation or go further into the level of Energy, where the patient describes qualities of the substance required, or can even name the substance directly. During the casetaking process, the patient may take the practitioner through the different levels of Emotion, Delusion, Sensation, or even Energy. The whole process of casetaking is divided into four steps, which are not fixed but more fluid. The steps tend to overlap each other.

In casetaking one should concentrate on the chief complaint, no matter whether the problem is emotional or physical. Do not assume that just because someone comes in with a physical symptom that is their main complaint, always ask them what is bothering them the most. The chief complaint is the main support around which the case revolves. In the old method, casetaking went all around the different areas of the patient's life, instead of catching hold of the chief complaint and not letting it go. But Sankaran and others found that what was clothed in the expressions of the emotional state becomes naked in the chief complaint. When the case is explored in the other areas first, only the tremors are felt. If the homeopath concentrates on the chief complaint right from the outset, then he discovers the volcano from where the tremors originate. If the focus is on the chief complaint, its sensation and modalities, then the very core of the case comes out right away.

The body and the mind both express the same phenomenon, the same disturbance, and the same vital problem. If the homeopath understands the physical aspect first (even if it is an emotional problem), it may save him from getting lost in the story. This new approach to casetaking was the beginning of an understanding of the various levels of perception and led to the discovery of the seven levels, Name, Fact, Feeling, Delusion, Sensation, Energy and Potentiality. The Seven Levels will be covered in detail in Unit Two.

The homeopath needs a lot of persistence, and no embarrassment in order to ask the same thing over and over again. When the homeopath understands all aspects of the case, he will see the same thing over and over, which is the Vital Sensation that connects the mind and body.

When the prescription is based on deeper levels it can be more effective. Taking the case according to levels of experience offers many advantages:

• The practitioner knows where he is in the casetaking process and how to proceed further;

• It defines what to look for and how to question further;

• The process of casetaking is more systematized.

Step One

Relentlessly Pursue the Experience of the Chief Complaint

The case begins by the practitioner asking for a detailed description of the chief complaint. He keeps asking the patient to describe it further and further until the patient comes to a sensation that has a greater connotation than just the physical problem. It is a good idea to usually stick to very simple questions at this stage, like "tell me more." For example, a woman comes with a pain in the upper left abdominal hypochondriac and is asked to describe the pain. She says, "This pinch thing is inside. I don't know where it comes from." The homeopath asks, "Please describe further." She says and gestures, "This pinch is like little bites, I can feel two three bites at the same time." The homeopath says, "Tell me more." She says, "…maybe like pins on the cloth, like my skin is pulling out." The homeopath reassures the patient and says, "You are explaining very well, please tell me more." She says, "I can feel this region is being attacked…"

The homeopath has to be relentless about pursuing the experience of the chief complaint and notice descriptive words that carry some intensity through gestures or intonation of the voice. It is essential to stick to the chief complaint and examine all its components thoroughly and exactly.

Bring the Patient Back to the Chief Complaint if he Diverts

If the patient shifts away from the description of the specific experience of the chief complaint, the homeopath must find a way to firmly bring them back to the experience of the chief complaint until it is completely described. One way to do this is to gently interrupt the patient, and repeat the last descriptive words and ask for a further elaboration of the experience. In the beginning of casetaking, if a patient diverts to some emotional aspects of his life, then bring him back to the chief complaint.

Acknowledge and Support the Patient through the Casetaking Process

It is usual for the patient to become exasperated and exhausted with the constant repeating of the same questions around their chief complaint. The homeopath has to be aware that the patient needs reassuring. A short explanation of the method can be helpful here, such as, "You have explained your experience very well, and each time I ask the same question you give a little more information, which helps me to understand your case." It is necessary to continually acknowledge that the client is answering the questions well, and that the practitioner is repeating the question not because he does not understand their answer but that each time they answer they give more useful information. For example, "You are doing great, I understand that the pain is sticking, poking, hard, please tell me more…."

Recognize Energy Patterns

The homeopath has to pay attention and recognize energy patterns during the patient's explanation of the chief complaint. For example, the person keeps describing a pinch and then with a strong hand gesture says bites. The homeopath must note this hand gesture and the word "bites." The practitioner needs to look out for repeated hand and facial gestures, and more generalized body language, until a pattern is recognized. At the moment the gesture is discovered, if the description continues to have consistency and energy, the practitioner should explore it further, for it can lead directly to the Vital Sensation.

In the previous example of the woman with a pinching pain, the homeopath knew he was close to the Vital Sensation because of the hand gesture and the intense intonation of "being attacked." From there the patient quickly jumped to a related image. She said, "I feel I am being attacked by some kind of worm." The idea is to see enough of the repeated energy (same gestures or intensity of words) so that the homeopath knows when to jump with a question to explore the image in depth, with as much detail as possible.

Observe Hand Gestures, Body Language and Intonations

With this method of casetaking, Sankaran realized that in many cases sensations were best expressed by hand gestures, even better than the words sometimes. The 'forced out' feeling of Liliaceae, the 'obstructed' feeling of Cruciferae or the 'pinched' feeling of Rosaceae can be well observed even when the words may actually be saying something else. These hand gestures are subconscious, involuntary and often not even noticed by the patient. Sometimes it is important to stop the patient while he is gesturing and ask him what the gesture means.

In one case the patient described her asthmatic attacks as a sensation of being tightly twisted in her upper chest, like choked or strangled. She gave a picture of the sensation like a python strangling its prey. Later on in the case she spoke of being hurt when her husband admonished her. When she was asked to describe the feeling of hurt, she used the word sad, while at the same time she clenched her hands and moved them towards her chest. It was the same gesture she used while describing the strangled and twisted feeling in the chest. She was unaware that her hands told us more than what she could express in words.

Hand gestures are important when they are repetitive in various different situations described by the patient and at different levels of the case. Pay attention to any gesture that is out of context with what is spoken. For example, the patient says, "I feel love" and gestures a clenched fist.

The practitioner can ask about the hand gesture specifically, when he is sure that he is at the level of Sensation, or when they are clearly repetitive.

What to Do if the Client Cannot go any Further with the Chief Complaint

If the homeopath confronts a case where the patient cannot elaborate further than the basic description of the chief complaint, the most useful next question would be: How does this chief complaint affect the patient's life? This often will open up another starting place for exploration, without deviating from the chief complaint. For example, a patient comes with a migraine and keeps repeating that it is a migraine, like a pain in the head, a migraine. The homeopath would then ask, "How does this migraine affect your life?" Then the patient might say, "It stops me from working at my best and paralyzes my social life." At this point the homeopath would continue to explore the effects of the chief complaint until the patient exhibits some intensity in the gesture, words or experience described. Then the homeopath can start to focus on the specifics of the experience, the words or the gesture.

The homeopath can discover: What does the chief complaint mean for them in their life? What does it stop them from doing? What problems does it create?

In another case the patient may express a specific modality, which the homeopath can ask the patient to explore further. For example, the pain is ameliorated by pressure. By exploring the feeling of the pressure, the homeopath can get closer to the Vital Sensation through the modality and its effects in the patient's life.

Often the patients will furnish more and more details about when and why the chief complaint happened. However, what the practitioner needs to know is what is happening. It is good to tell the patient that they have explained very well the situation, but what they experience is more important.

First Sensations Expressed by the Client May Not Be the Vital Sensations

The homeopath should not be deluded by the first expressions of a sensation from the patient about their chief complaint, because they might not be the Vital Sensation. It is only through a continuous exploration that the sensation can be confirmed through repetition, gestures, images, energy. For example, the patient comes with a pain in the knee and says he feels very tight and cannot walk. Now is this feeling of tight a local sensation or a general sensation? Try to understand the local sensation very precisely. Ask more about the local sensation. Where does it lead to? Probe the word or the gesture up to the point where it does not go any further or till the patient repeats images about the same thing. Be aware that the first thing a patient says about the sensation of his illness may not be the Vital Sensation. Just follow the lead till it leads to the Vital Sensation, or there are images, or the client cannot go any further.

Exploring Different Levels

When chasing the Vital Sensation, the client will travel through different levels of experiences of his perspective of the world, from the superficial to the deepest core. It starts from the diagnosis (Name level) and details of the illness (Fact level); then to the various related emotions (Emotion level); then to the metaphorical perception of these emotions (Delusion level). Further investigation leads us to the level of Sensation and energy patterns in the case. The Energy level is expressed as speed, color, sound and direction, and is non-human specific. The level of Sensation is the realm of raw experience. At the levels of Sensation and Energy are the likely places where the patient can give descriptions of the actual source material of the remedy needed. When the homeopath reaches the level of Sensation or raw experience, there he will find the Vital Sensation which will manifest throughout the patient's case and all the other levels.

For example, the patient says, "I am totally lost; I don't know what to do, I feel confused, bewildered." This Vital Sensation was confirmed because it was expressed at the level of Sensation in all aspects of this patient's life, dreams, physical reactions, work situations, relationships, hobbies, and so forth. This level of Sensation is recognized by the homeopath when it is expressed as raw experiences at all levels and not to be confused with the Fact level, which is local and specific to a particular area of the patient's life. For example, the patient says the pain is burning and achy, but has no other sensation of this type in the case. This sensation would be at the level of Fact.

The Level of Emotion

If the patient does not give you a clear cut local sensation or gives many sensations, then look for emotions, which are associated with the chief complaint. Then explore these feelings deeply. Try to see what is peculiar and how these emotions are perceived and experienced, which will help to arrive at the level of Delusion.

When the patient can only express an emotional feeling, the practitioner can ask: How does the client experience the feeling in the body? What are the physical symptoms he experiences at the time? This type of questioning often will lead toward the Vital Sensation.

By questioning the emotions, the homeopath can get to the level of Sensation, or what the patient experiences physically and emotionally when he is in that situation. For example, the patient may describe the emotion as a fear. Then the next question would be: "Where do you experience that fear?" or "How do you experience that fear?"

Images and the Level of Delusion

With persistent and focused questioning, there are two main ways the patient will express the level of Delusion. He could give a visual picture or an example. For example, if he says he feels stuck to one point and the homeopath persists with asking him to explain, the patient may say that he is stuck to one point as if he is in the middle of a street and there is a car coming at him at full speed… This is how he feels stuck in such a case. The second way the patient can reach the level of Delusion is by associating his chief complaint with something else in his life or in his story. For example, he can spontaneously describe an incident when he was going across the street and felt stuck in the same way.

Usually if the patient goes in depth into the description of the sensation of the chief complaint and persists in this area, the patient will lead the homeopath to all the significant areas of this life, like work, relationships and interests, and to the level

Delusion. However, if the casetaking process is not progressing to the level of Delusion, then the homeopath needs to inquire into areas where the patient will show the least amount of compensation and the delusion is best expressed. Some of these areas to explore are hobbies, interests, dreams, fears, most stressful situations and childhood.

During the process of exploring the level of Delusion, Emotion, Sensation or Energy, be aware of out of context or strange language the patient may use as it might be related to the source material of the remedy itself. For example, different patients used images such as: the cabbage metamorphosed (a butterfly case), worries percolated into private life (a Coffea case), the lizard felt sticky (a Drosera case). Repetitive dreams or images are also useful, such as the case with the recurrent dream of crossing the street like a rat (a rat case).

Level of Sensation and its Opposite Sensation

The pursuing of the chief complaint brings the main feeling or sensation, which can come from questioning the patient about the facts, the emotions or delusions from the chief complaint. The presenting problem can be seen as an expression of the Vital Sensation. The questions leading to the level of Sensation would be to find out about the situation, and then to ask: What is the experience of that situation? What is the feeling in that situation? What is the sensation?

Once the sensation is understood, then explore the opposite sensation, which is especially useful in identifying plant cases. Again the areas of least compensation (hobbies, interests, dreams, childhood), may bring out the opposite sensation, which may come up naturally or need to be investigated directly. For example, in a Mangifera case the patient needed to be in company. When she was asked about her feeling when in company, she replied that she feels things are moving and are not static. What does that have to do with company? This response fits with the rest of the case. Mangifera is a Sycotic remedy from the Anacardiaceae family. The main sensation in this plant family is of being caught or stiff or stuck. The opposite sensation was found in her hobby, where she was not static and always moving. The beauty of this casetaking method is that anything can come up; and as the case goes on the sensations and feelings unravel as a surprise.

Recognizing the Miasm

As the patient describes his chief complaint, the homeopath also needs to note the pace and depth of the problem, and the patient's response or attitude or coping mechanism, which indicate the miasm in the case. The miasm becomes apparent once the sensation is known and probed. When the homeopath sticks to the chief complaint and examines all the components thoroughly, the sensation and miasm are revealed. Miasms will be covered in depth in Unit Four.

Summary of Step One

1. The chief complaint is the central pillar around which the case revolves. It is the manifestation of the concentrated disturbance of the vital force at that moment. Pursue the chief complaint relentlessly.

2. At the beginning, simply ask the patient to tell more or to describe more.

3. Understand precisely the local experience of the chief complaint.

4. When the patient comes to the end of his ability to describe his chief complaint, ask how does the chief complaint affect the patient's life?

5. Pay attention to the description of the chief complaint: Does the patient express anything that is peculiar? How is it experienced? Is it experienced as a problem with structure, sensitivity or hierarchy? What is the level of experience?

6. Be aware that the language used to describe the experience of the chief complaint may help to indicate the kingdom of the case. For example, a local sensation may be expressed as an issue of sensitivity and reactivity, which may indicate a plant kingdom, while other sensations may give clues of the victim-aggressor issue (animal remedy) or issues of structure and function (mineral remedy).

7. Look for sensations, words or gestures that express energy and when questioned can lead further into the case.

8. Continue to reassure the patient, and acknowledge how difficult it must be, and explain that the purpose of this process is in order to get a good prescription for them.

9. Try to confirm the sensation through all the levels, and get the patient to describe the opposite sensation in detail, which may help the patient to spontaneously connect the sensation with images, situations, fears, or other aspects of his state.

10. The practitioner needs to have patience, endurance and faith that the patient will express something deeper and go to all the different levels in order to make an accurate prescription.

Important Rules to Follow

• Only use the words of the patient. Always repeat the same word in exactly the same way. Ask him to describe further, to tell more, and inquire about the sensation or feeling of the chief complaint.

• Keep asking the same question in various ways till the patient leads the practitioner to the next question or step. This is reached when the patient gives another clue or a sensation that is more precise or more descriptive or at a deeper level than the previous step.

Very Condensed Case to Illustrate Step One

[Sankaran's case and comments are edited from "An Insight into Plants, Volume 1." 'H' is the homeopath and 'P' is the patient.]

The patient is asked to tell why he is there.

>   P: Cough four to six times in the day. (Fact level)

>   H: Describe the cough some more.

>   P: I blank out with the cough…want of breath. I have a pulling sensation in the abdomen and throat. It is worse when I go out, from a draft of air…so I don't want to leave my home. It comes on suddenly, especially when talking.

It is possible to see that the patient has a cough which gets severe from time to time, and at such times he gets a blank out. The cough gets worse when he is outdoors and so he cannot go outside the house.

So there are two aspects to the cough:

• Blank out (local sensation);

• It comes from time to time and he can't go out of the house anymore (pace/miasm).

>   H: Tell me about blank out, please describe it.

>   P: It becomes black before my eyes, as if I am stuck to one point.

>   H: What does stuck to one point mean? What is the feeling when you are stuck to one point?

I have used only the words of the patient and keep up this questioning till he leads me to the next question. This could be a more precise feeling or a visual picture or something that comes up by association.

>   P: It is as if I cannot move.

Now this does not yield a finer description of being stuck at one point, nor has he given a picture of what it is like to be stuck at one point. You cannot go any further with this answer. So I will again ask about his feeling when he is stuck to one point.

>   H: What is the feeling when stuck to one point?

He reverts back to the chief complaint. Now it is our job to keep him on track so I repeat the same question till he goes one step deeper.

P: It is like you are in the middle of the street and a car is coming at full speed. That is how I feel.

Now this is a visual picture (level of Delusion). It could have been an actual experience from his life. It is a window into his mental state, which gives a deeper understanding than the physical complaint. Question him further and ask about his experience in this situation, and then the homeopath may be able to see a connection with the cough.

H: How does one feel when one is in the middle of the street and a car comes at you at full speed?

P: It happened to me as a child. I felt the same way.

It is important to get to the sensation in that situation. Ask him now to describe the experience in emotional and physical terms.

The case started with the cough, then came to blank out, then to black before the eyes, then to stuck to one point, and then to the childhood situation. All this information came by sticking to the chief complaint and chasing it.

P: The fear is I will be suddenly killed and so I cannot move.

So in this manner by chasing the chief complaint, the homeopath can come to the main feeling or fear which is that suddenly the patient feels he is going to be killed and he is stupefied from this fright. Now it is possible to see the connection with the cough. The cough comes suddenly from time to time and he cannot go out of the house. It gets black before the eyes and he is stuck to one point as if he is going to be killed. He is frightened and stuck to one point. Fright stupefies. The cough stupefies. He avoids going out of the house because he will get a cough. He avoids the situation that stupefies him, but he still gets the cough from time to time.

This case is from the Solanaceae family and from the malarial miasm, which would be the remedy Capsicum. The remedy became apparent from the chief complaint and was confirmed in other areas of the case.

Step Two

The next step in casetaking is to dissociate the patient from the local phenomenon (the chief complaint or situation) and to understand the Vital Sensation as a general sensation. In most cases the homeopath has to hold on to the energy by focusing on the repeated gesture or intense word, and the patient will generalize the sensation on his own. The questioning continues to follow the sensations until it is non-human specific. At this stage of the case the practitioner notes the pace, the depth and the degree of the problem, which are indicators for the miasm.

The sensation becomes general when:

• Experienced in the same way in another location other than the chief complaint, or

• Expressed through repetitive or intense gestures, or

• Experienced in the form of energy, which are non-human specific words or descriptions.

While exploring the general sensation, the patient may go back to emotions or images or may jump into the level of Energy (a non-human specific expression, such as break, tight, hot, etc.). Go back to the sensation that the patient has repeatedly confirmed and take the patient deeper till he gives a situation (actual or metaphorical) where the sensation, miasm and kingdom concur.

After finding the sensations and actions in the chief complaint, the next step is to confirm these findings in the areas of least compensation. The same sensation or its opposite, as well as the action, must be found in hobbies, dreams, childhood, and so forth. When the common sensation is confirmed in all these areas, then the core of the case has been reached and cannot be disputed. Now the homeopath can freely go into other areas, especially those that are seemingly disconnected and see how they connect to the common sensation.

All patients have features of all the kingdoms (plant, mineral and animal) and will use language from other kingdoms in a superficial way. The homeopath has to go to the most underlying basic structure to differentiate the kingdom. Is it a problem of survival (animal), structure (mineral) or sensitivity (plant)? This cannot be considered in a superficial way. It is important to go to the depth and find out how the problem moves them at that depth. What creates the turmoil in the patient? What will make the patient all right? This understanding has to be in every aspect of the case: dreams, chief complaint, and so on. The homeopath has to determine what kingdom the core state of the case lies in. It is also possible to consider the nosodes and the group of imponderables, which will not fit into these three usual kingdoms.

The determining of the kingdom comes after the complete exploration of the Vital Sensation, and assessing the language of the Vital Sensation in terms of the classifications of kingdoms. For example, the case is all about survival and aggression, so the patient may need an animal remedy and the practitioner needs to explore the sub-kingdom (mammals, insects, birds, fish, etc.) and the miasm. The other units will cover a detailed explanation of kingdoms, sub-kingdoms and their analysis.

It is important to note at which point in the case the local phenomenon becomes general or emotional, or at which point emotional phenomena become physical. This is the Vital Sensation, something that connects the mind and the body. The most stressful areas in the life of the patient will often times reveal the sensation, miasm and kingdom together.

When there is an intense emotional phenomenon, how is it experienced physically? When there is an intense physical phenomenon, how is it felt mentally? The patient will commonly express the common sensation in metaphors, in an intense situation or emotion, in dreams, interests, hobbies, fears, fantasies, and in any book, story, movies, television serials that come spontaneously to their mind. The patient will use a phrase such as, it is like…The practitioner can ask: How did it feel? How did you perceive it? What was the experience like? See how it connects with the chief complaint. Detach the patient from the human feeling and situation, and take them to the non-human, Sensation or Energy level (Vital Sensation). Sometimes the practitioner needs immense patience to take the patient from the level of Emotion to the Delusion level and further to the Sensation level, and beyond.

Once the practitioner chooses to take the "mineral" road, the next step is to find the sub-kingdom, meaning which line in the periodic table (natrum, kali, argentums, aurums, etc.) is being expressed here. The practitioner also needs to understand if there are one or two themes in the case. Then the practitioner tries to understand how that line (following many themes of Scholten and further explained by Sankaran) intersects with the Vital Sensation, and is expressed throughout the case. In the mineral cases when the practitioner recognizes if the patient needs a salt or a pure substance, and knows the line or lines of the minerals required, then the depth and intensity of the Vital Sensation will give the stage of the periodic table where the miasm is often identified. Then it is often important to confirm the remedy choice through the Materia Medica, and sometimes in the Doctrine of Signatures.

Once the practitioner chooses to take the "plant" road, then it is important to confirm that the Vital Sensation is persistent and repetitive. Often times there are consistent and opposing sensations, which continue to be reconfirmed throughout the case. The repeated sensations help to identify the sub-kingdom. The specific Vital Sensations have been charted in many of the plant families, which give the homeopath the possibility to easily identify the sub-family and then the specific remedy by identifying the miasm. The probing of the Vital Sensation at the level of Sensation will give the miasm, which will be explained in depth in Unit Four. For example, the specific common Vital Sensation is stuck, caught, motion ameliorates, which indicates the *Anacardiacea* plant family. The miasm is Typhoid, and then the homeopath will know to prescribe *Rhus-toxicodendron*.

Once the practitioner chooses to take the "animal" road, then he has to probe the Vital Sensation, for the intensity and depth in order to determine the miasm of the case. The recognition of the miasm will come from the exploration of the language of the Vital Sensation and will help to give the sub-kingdom (i.e. Tubercular miasm may be an insect remedy, Sycotic miasm possibly is a milk remedy, etc.) When the practitioner is in the sub-kingdom, he continues to explore the Vital Sensation until the patient gives enough qualities and language to confirm the specific animal remedy, which can be confirmed in dreams, hobbies, books, movies (anything that excites the person at the level of Delusion and Emotion).

Once the practitioner chooses to take the "nosode" road, then he can probe the Vital Sensation and the language of the miasm until it is repeated in all spheres of the case. For example, the patient is only speaking about the need to escape, can't breathe, needs to change continuously, and so forth, the prescription could be *Tuberculinum*. Be aware that the expression of the miasm must be consistent and intense in the case, and that none of the other kingdoms predominate.

The imponderables are an unknown territory. However, when a patient describes in specific language a substance that is an imponderable and its energy pattern is consistently expressed throughout the case, the homeopath can consider it for a prescription.

Step Three

Step three is a review of all the previous steps in casetaking. The case is complete if at every step the same sensation and energy pattern is unearthed. A word becomes a general phenomenon and can be confirmed when the experience is described vividly or emphasized again and again in all aspects of the patient's life.

For example, the patient says "I have a pain in the neck and feel very tight." The doctor asks, "What is tight?" He replies, "My neck becomes very stiff and I cannot move." The local sensation is tight, stiff, and cannot move. However, the practitioner has to examine how this tightness and stiffness is seen as a general phenomenon before deciding if the local sensation is the Vital Sensation. Once the Vital Sensation is clarified, then the homeopath should trace the sensation further until the kingdom, sub-kingdom and source are revealed.

Step Four

One of the goals of this method of casetaking is to take the patient to the point where they are using the language of the substance that is needed, for example: I am 360 degree, go into the ground, up in the sky and provide shade (sounds like a tree). More extensive explanations of stages three and four will be in Unit Five.

Upon completion of all four stages, the homeopath is ready to make the prescription.

A Sample List of Questions for Casetaking

Casetaking is like climbing down a ladder, each expression with energy is a rung to climb down deeper and deeper. A particular level is thoroughly examined until a firm footing is established before proceeding to the next level. Whenever the patient slips back, there is a gentle prodding onwards to go deeper.

It is necessary to keep the questions open ended so that the patient leads the way. The homeopath recapitulates what was said and asks the patient to continue on the path to express their state. The words repeated back to the patient are exactly the same ones used by the patient. In the beginning of the case it is more useful to find a number of characteristic words with energy than a single word to repeat back to the patient.

• Tell about the problem (*chief complaint*).

• What (*repeating the patient's same words exactly*) troubles you or bothers you right now?

• So out of all the things that cause you stress what is the thing that affects you the most?

• How does it bother you?

• Describe this (*repeating their last words exactly*).

• Describe it more.

• What is the sensation?

• How do you experience (*repeat three or four words the patient used to describe their situation or experience*)?

• How does it feel?

• Describe this (*repeating the patient's words*) feeling a little more.

• What is the sensation that (*repeating the patient's words*)?

• When you say (*their last words*), what do you mean?

• Describe the sensation of (*repeating the exact the words of the patient*).

• How does (*their word*) feel?

• What is (*repeating the exact words of the patient*)?

• Tell about this.

• What does it feel like?

- Describe the opposite of (*repeating the exact words of the patient*).

- How does it feel when you have to (*do whatever*)?

- And then?

- When don't you feel (*repeating the exact words of the patient*)?

- Tell me about it.

- What was the effect of the situation on you?

- What would you feel?

- You said it was like (*repeating the exact words of the patient*), what does that feel like?

- What is the sensation of (*the exact words*)?

- What did you feel in that situation?

- What would make you feel better in these situations?

- What would give you the most relief?

- What do you feel when you are (*doing this that relieves you*)?

- What kind of book would you read?

- What would be the effect?

- What was the feeling?

- What are your dreams?

- In the past is there anything unpleasant? Or especially pleasant?

- Any daydreams?

- What is the feeling like?

- What are the feelings involved?

- Describe the (*repeating the exact words of the patient*).

- How would the pain be? How would you feel it, experience it?

- What is the sensation?

- Describe *(the sensation)*.

- Describe this sensation more.

- Describe this *(description so far)*.

- What is the opposite?

- Please give an example?

- In what situation have you felt *(repeating the exact words of the patient)*?

- Tell me about the *(particular situation)*.

- Describe it more.

- Tell me more.

- What is the sensation it creates in you physically or emotionally?

- How does that feel?

- You have described your situation very well. I don't want any more information about you, but what is *(repeating the words used)*?

- What does *(a particular word)* mean?

F. SAMPLE CASES
By Melissa Burch, CCH

A Case of a Woman with Sinus Pain

Homeopath: So tell me what the problem is now? What is going on for you now?

Client: The thing is that my sinuses have not improved yet. They have not improved. The thing is, last night, in fact. . .you see, I took the remedy and then I really did not want to do anything else for 24 hours. I wanted to give it a full chance, because, you know, I do this and that and then I cannot even pinpoint and say, "Oh, this is not working." I wouldn't know, because I did not give it enough of a chance. So I didn't do anything. I just took steam and the whole day I was the same, but in the night it became extremely horrible. Like now, my head is not achy until I move it. And that is typical of my sinuses, particularly. But when I move my head, it aches like anything. It is like extreme pain in the center of my head, here, and more toward the left. But I would also say the center and left, like that (HG (Hand Gesture)). And it is really painful whenever I move. Like if I am lying down, it is painful twice: once when I sit down and once when I stand. And when I move, I feel extreme pain. And this continues. It continued yesterday, but in the night I was in constant pain on the left side, completely, like here (HG), and including my eye. Like a plate here, if you divided my head with a plate. It was hurting like nothing I've ever felt before. I've never had that pain.

H: So tell me everything about this pain. You're doing very well. Just tell me everything you can about this pain.

C: Yes. I still have it, in fact, that's why I didn't take a pain killer today because I was going to meet you and I have pain here—exactly here (HG). And yesterday this pain was like a plate, going through.

H: Like a plate?

C: Yes, like a plate. Like a full plate. Like if you cut my head from here to here (HG), the whole half of it was hurting. But not the other side. I have not felt much pain on the other side or anywhere else, even on the edge here. But in this plate, which includes my left eye, I felt extreme pain. Extreme.

H: What kind of pain?

C: Extreme. I've never had pain like that before in my life. It was very, very painful. Very, very, very, very painful. Extremely. I couldn't speak. I couldn't do anything. And then I took a pain killer. I took something to relieve that pain, and it did not work completely.

H: Tell me more. Use more words for this extreme pain. You said it's like a plate, that comes straight across from the eye. . .

C: Yes, from the eye to here (HG). In fact, yesterday I asked my husband to do some massage for me on my head. And the moment he pressed here (HG), my whole head was in pain, so I wouldn't allow him to press here (HG). So probably there's some liquid in the back of my neck here (HG). The moment he pressed here (HG), everything was hurting. It was horrible, the whole of it. The pain that I have now is more a superficial pain, like I don't feel so much inside. It's on the surface, on the top, on the left, and on the back here. I would not say that I feel it in the center. I would say that it's on the top, on the left a little bit, and on the back. But this pain I had last night was completely through. I don't know how to explain it better. I can just say that it was extreme. It was as if it was going to break off, this part of my. . .

H: It was going to break off?

C: Yes. That's the feeling I had.

H: It would break off, like how? What would happen?

C: I don't know. I just couldn't take it. I'm sure it would be less painful to die. I don't know how else to explain it.

H: You're doing very well. Just some more. You said it's like a plate.

C: I didn't say it's like a plate. I said if you have a plate here (HG), then whatever parts are cut by that plate are hurting. If you insert a plate, then whatever parts of my head which are touching the plate on this level would hurt; not the plate, but my head.

H: Like it's a line?

C: Yes, it's a line, it's true.

H: And from here to that line is what is hurting?

C: Yes, yes.

H: And then the pain is so horrible, it's like it could break off.

C: Yes, it's continuous. In my sinuses I don't have continuous pain, I don't have it. It's only if I move that I have pain. Like if I am just sitting like this and talking, most likely I will not have pain. But that pain was continuous.

H: You're doing great. So what would this pain feel like, that it's going to break off? You said it was so horrible, as if it could break off. . .

C: I don't know how to answer this.

H: Okay. We're going to do a new method. What we're going to do now is that I'm going to ask you the same question over and over. It's not because you're not clear. You're actually very clear.

C: Yes, but you know if I verbalize it more, it will just change.

H: That's what I want. It doesn't matter. We're going to go to a new level with this case, just with this pain. We're only going to focus on this pain and then we'll see where we go.

C: Okay.

H: So you're going to go into a state that you've never had to describe before. You're going to have to find new words, so this is going to take some time. If you close your eyes, you'll feel it, and you can tell me whatever comes to mind. Don't worry if it makes sense or doesn't make sense. You just tell me what comes to mind. Okay?

C: So, ask again.

H: Okay. So you said it's like breaking apart.

C: No, I felt it could break apart.

H: Could break. Good.

C: It wasn't breaking, that's the whole problem was that it wasn't breaking—it was right there. I wish it would break apart, but it felt like it was really going to bust my head and maybe have a hemorrhage. I don't know what. It was so painful. It was so painful; it was not physically possible to bear that pain. It wasn't physically possible to bear it. Childbirth for me was even so much easier. It's a pain I've never felt before. So much.

H: Okay. So, describe the pain. You're doing great. Just describe.

C: This kind of pain. I don't know, I would just say continuous pain.

H: And the problem was that it didn't break off.

C: Yes.

H: It was like. . .explain this again to me so that I can understand it better.

C: You see, the thing is that it was hurting, the whole plane. It was like my head was going to break in two, I felt. But no, it wasn't breaking, the pain was right there. At a point I thought, "Maybe it's going to do some more damage inside me." I don't know. But I really can't explain it any better than that, even if you ask me ten more times.

H: I'm going to ask you ten more times. You're doing great. Because each time I ask you, you will give me a little more information. So it's actually useful. Okay?

C: Okay.

H: So it's like more damage, you were worried that it would cause more damage inside. So tell me more about this.

C: I don't know. I just feel like it was nothing but what I explained before. I was telling you all this because I am a headache person. I get headaches. I used to get, as a child, headaches very often. But this kind of headache I don't remember. I might have had one a long time back, but in my memory, it's never been like that headache. Never. Especially not like that with the plate. I was in pain so much, so much, that I felt like I couldn't take it. Because I can take a lot of pain. I can take a lot of physical pain, I think. Like even with my broken knee and all, I was walking to the hospital. I can take a lot of pain. Generally, I can. Headaches, I cannot take so much. But this I took a lot because I didn't want to interfere with by using medicine. I was very clear, I don't want to. Because all of this effort that we have done together, it breaks off. So I was all the time waiting. And it came upon me, I could not wait. "If I don't take medicine now," I thought. I just felt like I wasn't going to live, it was like, "I might die." It was so painful. I thought maybe it would create some damage inside me, this pain. I thought that maybe it was a nerve hurting through and through (HG). And I was trying to think of how to relieve this nerve of its pain because the pain might create further damage. Because a pain is helpful. A pain might help you relieve your problem. Because I know that until I'm in extreme pain, I don't take an effort to solve it. But this kind of pain was more than extreme. And if it didn't stop, it might create damage. That's all I felt.

H: So you said it's like the nerve itself.

C: Yes, I felt. When I felt that, it was the moment my husband touched here (HG) and everything was hurting. So I knew that there were some nerves that were going somewhere. And that one of them, probably, was hurting like anything. Probably it was not the whole of the plate, maybe just one nerve which was going to all of those parts. But including my eye, to the back of my eye was hurting like anything. Even the whole thing, from here to here, and it stopped here (HG).

H: But you go like this (HG).

C: Yes, I go like this (HG). I start here and it goes to here. Or maybe I start here and it comes to here. And not here, of course (HG). From the back of my neck, here (HG), to the lower part of my eye. Behind here everything was pain. And maybe, normally, at the same time the left side or the center would be hurting also. But because of that extreme pain, I could not register any other pain.

H: And what was the fear of the damage? What was the damage that could be created?

C: What kind of damage could it cause? It could cause a brain hemorrhage. I don't know. I don't know. It could just burst, maybe, the nerve. I mean, what was it that caused it to hurt so much? I don't know. If I knew what the cause was, then I would imagine further what would happen.

H: What would you imagine then?

C: Well I just feel that maybe the nerve would burst open.

H: It would burst open?

C: Yes. And create something like a hemorrhage, probably. But, of course, that was my imagination.

H: Can you tell me more? So it was coming through like this, like a nerve. If it got too bad, your fear was that it would burst.

C: Yes.

H: Any more? What exactly would the pain feel like? I still don't understand exactly. How would you describe this pain? I know it's so horrible, but what is the quality of this pain? It's as if. . .what?

C: I am trying to think as if what. It's as if what? I don't know. I've never felt anything like that before and this pain itself I've never felt before. I don't know.

H: But you felt it last night.

C: Yes.

H: And it was so horrible. And you had the feeling that it could break apart, like split you in two.

C: I mean, I wished it would.

H: You wished it would, okay. Exactly. And that it might cause some damage. That it might burst and cause damage and hemorrhage or something like that.

C: Yes, yes.

H: But what is the quality of the pain?

C: What's the quality of the pain. . .it's like what. . .(pause) it's like an earthquake.

H: It's like an earthquake. Good. Very good.

C: With a crack in the middle. And the whole line.

H: Cracking in the middle. With a line. Great. Okay, so tell me everything you know about earthquakes and cracking in a line like that. Not so much the headache, okay? You made it very clear what happened in that situation. But tell me everything you know about earthquakes and cracking in a line like that.

C: Probably so much pressure in the head that it creates an earthquake. So much pressure. The pressure could be because of some psychological reason or it could even be the pain itself. The pressure caused by the pain itself. Yes, that's the pain I felt. The pain and the pressure. A lot of pressure. In a sense that I couldn't avoid it. Of course, any pain you cannot avoid, but this one was completely like that (HG). Like can I tell you now that my head is hurting in the center and in the back. But that time I couldn't even feel that because this was hurting so much more.

H: Very good. So tell me everything you know about this kind of pressure, like an earthquake with a cracking line. Not you, because you've described yourself very well. Now I just want you to tell me what this kind of experience would be like, not so much with your headache, but just, what is this kind of so-much-pressure like an earthquake that's cracking in a line?

C: Yes, I am trying to understand. One thing is that it is not just a line; it's like that (HG). It's a crooked line, not a straight line. That's what occurs to me when I talk about an earthquake. Another thing that occurs to me is that there is a definite distinction between the crust of the earth and something that it going to come out from the inside. There's a definite distinction between the crust, which is cracking, and what is going to come out, which is completely different.

H: What is it that comes out?

C: What comes out is kind of a liquid, a solid liquid. Kind of a lava. Like that. Not lava exactly, what I feel. I do not associate it with lava; I associate it with something very soft, but not solid, not liquid. Like a jelly.

H: Like a jelly?

C: Yes, coming out.

H: Okay, what is this jelly that's coming out?

C: It has a solid mass, although I would say it's like rubber. Soft and hard at the same time. Yes, that's all, soft and hard at the same time. If you ask me to imagine, it's more transparent, with the illusion of color. But that's my imagination.

H: I want your imagination, you're doing beautifully. Very good. So, it's jelly-like, but it's more rubber.

C: Yes. It's a jelly, but not like a jelly that you eat, because it's like rubber (HG). It's transparent and light yellow in color. And it does not have any property of the earth.

H: Meaning?

C: Meaning the earth, which was cracking, is completely different. And what is coming out is completely different.

H: Well, what's coming out? Tell me more about what's coming out.

C: I feel really funny.

H: This is good. You're doing perfectly. This is exactly what I need. You're doing just perfectly. So you said it's like rubber, it has this kind of quality like. . .

C: Yes, but it's continuous. It's not coming out in one single motion like that (HG). It's all continuous throughout the crack. Throughout the crack, it is continuous and coming out at the same time (HG) and round. Not coming out like water, but coming out like this (HG). This is how I am imagining it.

H: Good. Okay. What else? Tell me everything you can see with this, that it's coming out like this (HG). It's rounded. . .

C: It's coming out cylindrically, throughout the length. Yes, and I don't want it to come out.

H: You don't want it to come out? What happens if it comes out?

C: I want to stop the earth from cracking, basically.

H: And tell me everything you can about the quality of this thing that's coming up from the earth, through this crack.

C: I'm imagining it is something very swollen inside my head.

H: No, no. Go back to the earth. Everything you can tell me about this. It's light, transparent yellow. It's round. And it's coming up from the crack, everything. . .

C: It's not round, it's a cylinder.

H: A cylinder, good.

C: It's long, so it can't be round. It stops like that (HG). But inside, I don't know what shape it has. When it's coming out, it's round, but inside is continuous with the earth. It is joined, literally, with the center of the earth. So when it's coming out, you can only see that part. What it's like inside, I don't know. But, it can't come out.

H: And what's it's temperature? Does it have a smell?

C: No, I don't feel any temperature. I don't feel that it is cold or hot or anything. It's a normal, room temperature, I would say. Because when you asked me what I was imagining, I said lava. But, I said, no, it's not lava, because it's not hot. Other qualities, I feel it's very innocent.

H: It's very innocent, okay. And innocent means what?

C: I would say innocent means something that is not damaging.

H: It's not something damaging.

C: No.

H: Okay.

C: It's not something damaging, but it has a quality which mucus has. You know, the quality that you don't want it.

H: So what is it that you don't want?

C: The rubbery aspect of it, maybe. I don't know. It's slimy. Kind of sticky. Not really sticky, but I don't know how to explain this. There is something about it that relates to mucus, which I don't like.

H: Very good. You're doing really, really well. It's very clear. So more about this rubbery aspect. More about the qualities of this rubbery aspect you don't like. It's slightly sticky, but not really sticky.

C: No, it's not sticky. It's not really sticky. If you touch it, it's not sticky. But it has this kind of elasticity (HG). Maybe if I break it, it will be like a jam.

H: If you break it, it's like a what?

C: If you take a spoon out of it, maybe it would be like jam, like sticky inside. You know when you take some part of jam, it sticks on the rest, so the inside of it is like that (HG). So the sticky property is inside, not on the surface of it. And that is maybe what I don't like about it.

H: And where else would you see this? Because you said it's not really like lava, it's room temperature. But it has something that comes through a crack like that.

C: Yes, yes.

H: What else could come through a crack like that that might be similar to this?

C: That's a very interesting question, only I can't think so much right now.

H: You're doing very well, so just. . .

C: What else could come out like that?

H: Or more qualities you can think of for this. It has a smell, or no smell?

C: Actually, I don't have the perception of smell. Did you know that?

H: No.

C: Did I not tell you?

H: No. Never, or. . .

C: Very high smells. Very, very intense smells I get. Like I can't smell any perfume. I can't smell any flower.

H: And this is just since when?

C: Ever since I realized I cannot smell. I was 15, I think, when I realized I can't smell. Because before that I used to imagine smells. And then I realized I could not make a distinction between a rose flower and any other flower. That's because I couldn't smell. I tried to smell different things and I couldn't smell. But my taste is not related to it, because I can taste, but I can't smell. But like petroleum, I can smell at the gas tank. So that kind of a smell, I have.

H: If it's very strong, then you can smell it.

C: Yes, because somebody told me to try eating fish, and after, I could smell better. I could smell more things when I started eating fish. And somebody told me it's because of a lack of zinc in my constitution. But I've not really worked further on it. So I would not be able to smell this thing that you're asking me, because it's not a part of my perception.

H: So what other qualities? It's bright yellow, it's a bit like the jam.

C: Brownish yellow. Sometimes it's light yellow, sometimes it's brownish yellow.

H: And it comes like. . .can you help me describe it?

C: Like honey. It's like honey.

H: So what is it that's like honey?

C: The color is like honey. The transparency, like honey.

H: And it comes through a crack.

C: Yes.

H: But it's not lava.

C: What else could come out from a crack? I don't know. I'd have to give it a lot of thought to know what else could come out from a crack like that. Like I'm sure there must be something that I'm relating to, but I don't know.

H: But you said it's like mucus, you relate it to the mucus in your nose from the sinus problem.

C: Yes. Because it's. . .

H: Because what?

C: Because of the stickiness of it inside, but not outside. Because of that.

H: But how does it come out? You said it comes out in a line?

C: Yes. There's a full crack, and it's coming out everywhere. It's coming out everywhere, and with this kind of a surface (HG) on the top. Not like water, like mercury. Mercury has like that (HG).

H: And how is it similar to mercury or different?

C: No, no. Nothing. Mercury I don't know.

H: Just the way it's coming out rounded like that.

C: Yes.

H: Okay. I have some ideas.

C: I'm sure I will relate it to something, but I can't recollect now what it could be. What could come out from a crack like that? What is the crack doing?

H: That's a good question. What is the crack doing?

C: A crack to me is a crack in a relationship. Generally that's a crack. Otherwise, what? Otherwise in the earth itself. Like too much of settled earth causing cracks, even those are the cracks that could relate too.

H: What else? Very good.

C: Because I know there are cracks in the feet, there are cracks in the cups and all. But what amazes me more are the cracks in relationships.

H: So tell me about this crack in the relationship.

C: I already told you the other day.

H: I know, a little more.

C: I don't know whether I should say this. I'm not so open about my husband as I was. Before when I started coming to you, I didn't have any practice and I thought I must open my head and tell you everything. But I don't know you enough to tell you all my life.

H: But you know this is completely confidential.

C: I know, but I should feel like talking. I don't mind you telling twenty people, that's not my problem. My problem is, I should feel like talking. And half the time I feel like I don't have to press myself to talk.

H: But you've done so well here and you're almost there. But do you know how it works? When you use the words that you used for the pain, then you use them for your emotional life, and the it's very important that they connect.

C: I know. I'll try.

H: Because this is probably why you got this headache. You said you never had something like this before.

C: I have been having sinus problems. This is the third time. But not so much pain.

H: But you said you don't remember this kind of pain. And now you're in a new situation. You didn't have this problem before.

C: But this is the first time I didn't take a pain killer. And I allowed the pain to go up.

H: And now we have a clear image. You gave a beautiful description. But for me to confirm, then, if I hear how you relate to it in your emotional life, then I know for sure we are on the right track. Anyway, I think you described it very well. But sometimes the words you will use in the relationship will relate to what we need to find for you. So I'm listening with a different kind of listening, you know.

C: Okay, I'll tell you.

H: So it must be connected, because this happened quite suddenly. And this situation is quite new for you.

C: Yes.

H: So somehow they are very connected. And you used the same words.

C: Yes, they are very connected. I know they are connected.

H: Okay, you tell me the connection.

C: Yes. I see a crack in our relationship. I don't feel like talking about it (tearfully).

H: Just tell me what a crack means. You don't have to say about the relationship, it's okay. But just tell me what this crack means. You said that it's a crack, that if I was somebody who didn't know any English at all, and you had to describe. . .do you want me to get you some tissues?

C: Yes.

H: So more about this plane, huh? You said that it is like on the earth. Just more about the plane. Not so much in the relationship, but what is plane? What are other images of a plane?

C: I just see the earth. But what you see for earth might be different from me, so let me just explain. By earth I just feel like this normal brown soil that we see. That's the kind of earth I imagine. Something quite stable. Very stable. Which is cracking. And I can see the crack.

H: And why is it cracking?

C: Why is it cracking? You want to talk about the earthquake, right, and not my relationship at all?

H: Just stay with this earth that's cracking. What might be causing this cracking?

C: It was the time, maybe. Maybe just the time.

H: Meaning what?

C: I don't know why the earth has cracked. I can only see it crack. I cannot see it before how it was. I can't make that determination as to why it cracked.

H: So you said that it's whole and not cracked. And then it cracks.

C: No, I just see it cracked.

H: You just see it cracked, okay.

C: Yes, I don't see it as a whole. I'm just looking at the two parts and telling you what it looks like, but it doesn't look whole to me.

H: And what's coming out is transparent, yellow, room temperature, and coming out from the earth.

C: I don't feel a temperature at all. I mean, I don't know even if it is room temperature.

H: And it's coming up how fast or slow?

C: Slowly. But it's going up.

H: And then what happens to it?

C: It's only a few feet down from the top of the earth. It's going out, I can see it.

H: And then what happens when it comes out?

C: It like will go on one or both of the sides of the earth. But I don't know what will happen later, because I can't see it. Do you only want to know about the severe pain that I have and not the general pain that I have with my sinuses?

H: You have that now, this general pain?

C: Yes.

H: Okay, yes. Tell me more.

C: Like it's on the left of the head, on the top and on the back. And whenever I move, it hurts like anything. It hurts like as if. . .how does it hurt? It hurts like some water, if it is still and you shake it. The kind of movement it creates, it creates in my head every time I move. It's extremely painful. Extremely. The only reason why I can suffer it is because it's not constant. It only happens when I move, so I try not to move. But if I cough, it's horrible. It's like water being shaken from the center. It's horrible. It's horrible, this pain.

H: So more about this. . .what is this pain that's like water being shaken?

C: Yes, I was just trying to imagine how it hurts, because it hurts with every movement. So I imagine it as simple, calm water, but with every movement, it is given a blow from below. And then it shakes. It shakes with a lot of ripples. And it's extremely painful. That's how I feel it. When I cough, I feel like it's a blow from below. When I stand up, I feel like it's turbulent (HG). Like it creates an imbalance. That's how I feel.

H: So, again, let's take it not to the pain, because you've described the pain very well, with this water. But if you had to describe it without using your head as the source of the pain, what would be this water that's shaking. How would that be, that situation? Can you describe that more?

C: I just see it as tranquil water that's disturbed. And when it's disturbed, it is getting too disturbed. It's not like if you disturb some water a little. It's too much disturbance. Too much. It's like. . .like that (HG).

H: Like that (HG)?

C: Yes.

H: So, what's this (HG)?

C: Ripples on the water.

H: So, more about these ripples on the water. What are the qualities. . .everything you can tell me.

C: Yes, it's very strong water, like the sea water. Not soft water like we get in the tap—hard. Hard water, and dark blue in color, I would say. Dark blue, but also, this water has the quality of having different colors. So not dark blue like a dark blue paint, but water that is dark blue or dark green, or maybe both from time to time. Very dark, actually. Very dark. It has all the properties of water, like it is liquid, it can create ripples. But ripples which are not calm ripples. Very up and down ripples. You know, like throwing a big stone in the water. Like that. Not throwing little pebbles, throwing a big stone in the water, and then the way it quakes. It's like that. That's how I feel.

H: And other properties? You said it's very, very dark.

C: Yes. It's very dark. It's almost transparent. It's on a tray. I imagine it on a very dark, almost black, tray. It's almost black, but it's not black, I think. It's on a very tilting tray, this water, and whenever there is an imbalance, there are lots of ripples. And it is painful.

H: And how does this relate to the other crack we talked about earlier?

C: It doesn't relate, in fact. Because when the water is stable, it doesn't hurt. It's only when it's not steady that it hurts. But the other crack was hurting continuously. So in a way, I don't see any relation.

H: You don't see any relationship?

C: No. Except that both are unbearable. Like when my head aches, you should see me, my face looks completely terrorized.

H: What is this terrorized look?

C: Just if you looked at my face at that time, you would think, "This lady must be in some kind of terror." Either in some terror or in some excruciating pain. You know, the pain which comes from seeing something which is very horrible.

H: Like what?

C: Like maybe a dead body. For me that is horrible enough. A face I would make like that would be the face when it's aching. But my face becomes like that because of the pain, not because of any feelings. It's only the pain. Physical pain, not emotional.

H: So what would it be like, all of this, what is this like? I mean you described it very well, but you have this thing that's so horrible, that it's like seeing a dead body. Can you say more about what this is like for you?

C: When I have this pain, I remember all kinds of gods and goddesses that I ever knew. When it hurts, it just reminds me of all the gods I ever knew. You know, it's so painful.

H: What does that mean?

C: That means I need help. I feel like I need help. I can't go on like this. I feel like I need help.

H: And what's that like, to need help?

C: Somebody to help me get rid of this pain. A pain which I know cannot be taken away instantly, because I know that it is my sinuses and it will take a couple of days to go, at least. So I need somebody to help me out of it. Not immediately, but at least to reduce the intensity of the pain. Meaning, I don't think you need something like a strong pain killer, but you just reduce the pain. I want the cause to also go away. That's very clear. Because pain is the outcome of the cause.

H: This is quite right. We have to find the part that is troubling. And somehow it's not something common. Otherwise we would have found it easily. We're having to find something quite special, which takes more time.

C: Okay. So, the last time my husband and I quarreled, it was on a different plane. I never had this feeling before, it was the first time. And for the first time, I see that we are on different sides, maybe on a badminton court. We are not on the same side like before.

H: So you're describing this rift in your situation very well, but what is rift then? What are other ways to describe this rift? You've described it very well, how you feel like you're on two sides of the badminton court.

C: Yes, and the net is the most important thing.

H: Why is the net the most important thing?

C: Because the net is what decides the two sides.

H: And what does that mean?

C: You can't go to the other side until you either go under the net or take it out. So you have to deal with the net first. And also that somebody else might lose if you win. That's something that happens if you're on opposite sides. Because until now, I always felt that my husband and I were on the same side. If one won, the other won also. If I won, he won also. It was like both of us were on the same side. But now I feel it's not like that. We are on opposite sides. So one winning, might mean losing for the other. And that creates a lot of difference between us.

H: And you said this net is the most important part. So tell me more about this net.

C: The net is very transparent, first of all. You can see each other, you can see everything. But you can't avoid it—it's there. And you have to deal with it. That's the net. So you can say it's transparent, but so what. You still have to deal with it. That is for me what net is. And the net is the one that defines the two sides. Otherwise there wouldn't be two sides.

H: It defines two sides. So just tell me about that. Outside of your situation. What is this defining two sides? What does that mean?

C: It defines two sides which could be similar. Like when I see a badminton court or a volleyball court, the two sides are very similar, so you can't say that this is good or that is good. But the fact that the net is there divides the two into separate parts. And come what may, they are not the same sides, they are different. And even if they are both good, even if they are both correct, they are two different sides. And separate.

H: And what does it feel like, to have two sides like this?

C: It's very depressing. It's a hopeless feeling. I realized that what keeps me going on is hope. Always hope and a dream. Because even if today I am not in a good place, tomorrow I'll be in a better one. I always had that hope for a better life, which I see crushed with this rift. I don't see any hope. I don't see hope. I don't see beautiful dreams anymore. And I think for me, when my dreams are crushed, I am crushed. Otherwise I am not crushed. That's also why I can't deal with death. Because death is something final that you can't change. I have heard beautiful stories about psyche and I have been reading that psyche never dies, but there's something that dies. The link dies. When a person dies, the bond which you have created dies. There is no way you can create that bond again. That's why I can't deal with death. And another thing that I can't deal with is hopelessness. It's similar to death.

H: You said it's like the bond dies. What is this bond? Tell me more about this bond that dies.

C: This bond is like a thick rope connecting people. But I don't give much thought to it, actually, in the physical sense. You want me to give thought to it right now?

H: Yes.

C: The bond. . .sometimes it's like this is shape (HG). And maybe like the shape of tendons. So for me, somehow the bond is also like that. More in the center, or maybe having a hole in the center, but that's how the bond is. Or sometimes like a tube, yes, with a similar material to what I saw in the crack. It's a similar material, but a different color. But I can't tell right now what color, because I'll just imagine any color and tell you any one that makes sense.

H: That's okay. Whatever first comes to your mind is fine.

C: The first color that came to my mind is like a darkish brown. Reddish brown.

H: How big is this tube?

C: How big is it?

H: Yes.

C: Not very big, like this (HG).

H: It's alive or it's not alive.

C: Right now I see it like it's in a glass tube. I don't know what that means. But it's constrained I would say. And right now I see a bar like that (HG), like a tube. A glass tube.

H: It's like a glass tube.

C: With this material inside. But this is what I see now. I didn't see it before.

H: It's good. So you have a glass tube with this inside. It's constrained. What else?

C: I can't seem to know more about the bar except for at the edges, the glass tube opens up at the edges (HG). That's all.

H: What's this (HG)?

C: The glass tube. When the cylinder opens up, it opens in little rectangles.

H: Can we go back to the thing that you said was so horrible. What is the experience for you emotionally with this?

C: Emotionally.

H: Yes. You've told me a little bit, but just a little bit more to understand this pain.

C: Yes, emotionally I feel that I've never been through this kind of pain before. That's what I feel.

H: And what's that like to have never been through such horrible pain?

C: It's like to have never gone through horrible pain like this before. . .

H: But you've gone through this, so what's it like to have gone through that pain?

C: I don't know. I don't know how to describe it.

H: Just emotionally what it was like for you to have been through that?

C: That's all I can say, that I never felt I've been through that much pain before. I've never been through that much pain before. I was in extreme pain, which I never was in before. In a way, now that we've talked so much, I feel saying, and it may be true, it may not be true, that I had many problems before, but not like this. That's the kind of feeling I had.

H: And problems like this, what. . .

C: I had many problems in my life which gave different kind of pains to me, but not so much pain as the feeling I had. That's what comes to me after talking so much about these things.

H: A little bit more. I know you've described these things very well, but a little bit more about what the experience of this pain is like for you. Just a little bit more. You've done really well, actually. Just a little bit further.

C: I don't know what to say.

H: Just a little bit more about what the experience of this pain was like for you. Just a little bit more.

C: Maybe you could rephrase the question and something else will come to me. Right now nothing else is coming to me.

H: So you said this was the most horrible pain, you've never been through something like this. This was the worst.

C: Yes.

H: What was it like for you to go through this? Just, if you had to tell someone, "I went through this horrible pain and it was like. . ."

C: Yes, I can say something. If my daughter wasn't here, I wouldn't have minded dying instead of having this pain. But because she is here, I would not think of dying. But, yes, I felt like I would rather die than have this pain. But, of course, I will not die because I have my daughter. So I will deal with the pain. That's the feeling I had.

H: So somehow, I'm jumping around a little bit, but somehow inside this tube is this brown thing and inside it was something like this substance that you described. And it was brownish red.

C: More liquid.

H: More liquid inside. And then when it came out?

C: No, it didn't come out. That's completely different. The only similarity between this and that was the kind of material.

H: Inside.

C: Yes. The kind of material, the property. The honey kind of property. I know why I remember honey—it's because of it's smoothness, because of it's color, because of it's transparency, and because of the fact that inside it is sticky. And I still don't feel the taste, whether it is sweet or not. I just see it like honey. Like a very smooth external surface with honey inside.

H: You have done very well.

Overview: Client is in an acute with extremely painful sinus headache and talks very fast. Great example of all levels all the time, which is common in acutes. Stays at fact level with headache pain then opens to source and connects with emotional pain which again goes to source.

Chief Complaint: sinus headache

Vital Expression: pain

Some questions the homeopath asks, once VE is identified:
What we're going to do now is that I'm going to ask you the same question over and over. It's not because you're not clear.
We're going to go to a new level with this case, just with this pain.
So you're going to go into a state that you've never had to describe before. You're going to have to find new words, so this is going to take some time. If you close your eyes, you'll feel it, and you can tell me whatever comes to mind. Don't worry if it makes sense or doesn't make sense.
I'm going to ask you ten more times. You're doing great. Because each time I ask you, you will give me a little more information. So it's actually useful.
And what was the fear of the damage? What was the damage that could be created?
Okay, so tell me everything you know about earthquakes and cracking in a line like that. Not so much the headache, okay?
So tell me everything you know about this kind of pressure, like an earthquake with a cracking line.
What is it that comes out?
Okay, what is this jelly that's coming out?
I want your imagination, you're doing beautifully.

Kingdom Language: plant, mineral
It was like my head was going to break in two ...I thought, "Maybe it's going to do some more damage inside me." I don't know. But I really can't explain it any better than that, even if you ask me ten more times.
Well I just feel that maybe the nerve would burst open
So much pressure
Death is something final that you can't change - When a person
dies, the bond which you have created dies. There is no way you can create that bond again

Source Language:
There is a definite distinction between the crust of the earth and something that it going to come out from the inside. There's a definite distinction between the crust, which is cracking, and what is going to come out, which is completely different.
It's coming out cylindrically, throughout the length
What comes out is kind of a liquid, a solid liquid. Kind of a lava... something very soft, but not solid, not liquid. Like a jelly.
It's a jelly, but not like a jelly that you eat, because it's like rubber (HG). It's transparent and light yellow in color
It's a normal, room temperature, I would say. It's not lava, because it's not hot.

It's not something damaging, but it has a quality which mucus has. It's slimy. Kind of sticky

It's like honey.

I know why I remember honey—it's because of its smoothness, because of its color, because of its transparency, and because of the fact that inside it is sticky.

Right now I see it like it's in a glass tube.

Energy Language:

Brownish yellow. Sometimes it's light yellow, sometimes its brownish yellow.

There's a full crack, and it's coming out everywhere. It's coming out everywhere, and with this kind of a surface (HG) on the top.

Miasm:

Extreme. I've never had pain like that before in my life. It was very, very painful. Very, very, very, very painful. Extremely. I couldn't speak. I couldn't do anything

I feel like I need help. I can't go on like this. Somebody to help me get rid of this pain. (Typhoid)

Remedy: terebinthinae oleum

Dose: 200c

A Case of a Woman with Pinching inside her belly

Homeopath: What the main things are then?

C: I have a pinch on my belly here (HG (hand gesture)) that is really worrying me. It is here, on my side, when I have my period. This thing pinches me in my side. I also have issues in my throat and a kind of cough, which keeps me from being able to sleep through the night. I wake up and 2:00 am and 4:00 am and 6:00 am. I wake up and then I go to the bathroom, then I drink some water and go back to sleep again. And when I work too hard I feel something here in this area of my foot (HG) which is very painful.

H: Just on the right foot?

C: Yes, mostly on the right side, but it can sometimes be on the other foot too. I also have numbness in my fingers when I hold something for too long. Finally, I would like to lose weight.

H: That's it.

C: Yes.

H: Of all these things, the pinch in the belly, this cough, being unable to sleep, and the pain on your foot, losing weight…what of these is the most troubling to you?

C: The most troubling to me, I think, is this pinch thing inside. I don't know where it comes from.

H: Okay, so tell me everything you can about this pinch.

C: This pinch, I don't know if it is some kind of worm, or if it is because I eat too many sweet things.

H: It could be a worm because of the sweet things?

C: Yes, but right now I'm not eating many sweets. But still, and I don't know why, but when I had my last period I started to feel the pinch inside. So, I don't know.

H: Okay, describe exactly the feeling of this pinch.

C: This pinching is like little bites, you know, like that (HG). And the bites cover a region, because I can feel two or three bites at the same time. So I don't know, it's very uncomfortable.

H: So it's like little bites, just tell me more about this, anything you can…

C: It's something at the side, here. It just comes and stays a little bit and then goes off.

H: So it stays a little while and then goes off.

C: Yes.

H: What I'm doing now…because you've described very well exactly the pinching and the little bites, and how it comes and goes, how it used to come
with your period, and now it just comes. So each time I ask you the same question, it's not because you aren't explaining it very well. It's just that every time you will tell me a little bit more. So that's why I'll keep asking you the same question, then we'll get more and more information. So just tell me again, it comes and it stays and then it goes off, what else can you tell me about it?

C: It comes and it pinches inside, little bites, maybe like the pins, like when you put pins on cloth, this kind of thing. And I'm not sure, but this time, I really relate it with my period.

H: So it's like pins on the cloth. Just, how do you experience these pins on the cloth?

C: I just think my skin is, it's like pulling out (HG).

H: Good, this (HG). Just, not this problem you have, because you described really well, just what is this pulling out? As much as you can use more words…

C: Just like little, little, bites.

H: Like little bites, like what kind of bites?

C: Let me see, I describe like bites, but I don't know, maybe it could be a pinch...

H: Bites it fine, you described it perfectly; it's not that, okay?

C: Alright.

H: What I'm looking for is more words. What would be the opposite of this pinching and these bites?

C: I don't know, I think that it is inside, but this thing comes and maybe it's some kind of alert.

H: Alert, like what kind?

C: It could be in my mind, but I think maybe it could be some kind of cancer. I could describe it like that. It is just a lot of pinching.

H: You said it's like an insect bite, it's like pinching; you feel it could be cancer; the feeling is there that it could be cancer.
C: Yes, because I feel the region is a circle, where they attack me. And it's not here or here and there (HG), it's just right here.

H: So it feels like it is one circle being attacked. Tell me about this. What is this attacked, just this one circle? It doesn't have to be this, just whatever comes to mind.

C: It's just, I feel this something underneath, like needles that come in and bite me.

H: Very good. It's like it comes in, it's like a needle, but it does this bite thing, it's like cancer, but it's an attack.

C: Yes.

H: No, I'm not saying that...we're in the realm of imagination, you don't need to worry. No, this is just to explore what your idea is.

C: Yes, this is my idea.

H: Very good. It's excellent. You are giving it perfectly. So now just explain to me more about this feeling that comes: it's like sewing, it's like biting, it feels like it could be cancer, that it is an attack...

C: Or it could be some kind of worm. Some kind of worm because in Brazil we check it out to see there are worms very quickly. And then we just take a little pill which makes you go to the bathroom and that's it. It's some kind of cleansing thing. But here I told the doctor and he said it could not be worms because people don't get worms here.

H: Tell me a bit more about how you experience it, what is it like for you to have this thing here that is like a circle...

C: Like I need to press my hand on it and I need to smooth the skin. And take the warm palm of my hand on top of it.

H: So it helps if you do that, if you go and you rub, and it's warm, and it feels better.

C: Yes, but it just comes and goes.

H: But how do you feel when this comes? It comes; it feels like a bite, it feels like this sewing, you described it perfectly. What is it like for you to have this? You said it could be cancer, in your mind, it could be worms.
C: I feel like I need to take better care of my body, to do some cleansing, and to do some limitation.

H: Limitation, meaning?

C: Limiting my food intake.

H: I'm going to go back. Because you've done beautifully, alright? It's not you, you've done really beautifully, it's just that I'm taking you to a place you've never had to go before. So that's why it will feel quite strange. But actually, you went very quickly, so we'll just go. This feeling, this pulling this biting, I'm going to take you back. Even just close your eyes and just describe with as many different words as you can what the sensation is, how this feels for you. It doesn't have to be exact; whatever comes to mind is really good.

C: What I feel is that there is something strange in my body. Like I'm growing something different there.

H: Good. Very good. So what does it mean to have something strange in your body, and something different? We're in the imagination, because you already explained it so well, exactly what it is, how it feels, when it comes. So now we're in the realm of imagination so it doesn't matter if it makes sense or anything. So what is this something strange in the body? Just whatever comes to mind. And it's growing, you said it's growing.

C: Yes, growing, because it doesn't stop. It comes and it goes off, so it is really something unusual. So this feeling is like, like little hands or fingers that go there and try to bite my meat or some part of my body. Something like that.

H: Okay, so it's biting. What could this be that's biting like this, just in the imagination, whatever comes? What is this that could be biting like this?

C: What could be biting? I don't know.

H: Just if you had to imagine, what would bite like this?

C: I think they are hungry or they want some sweets, or something. And if I don't appease them, they come and they give these bites.

H: Very good. Okay, what could be hungry that wants sweets and then gives these bites? What is it that could do that?

C: Could you ask me again?
H: What is it, in you imagination…okay, because you've used it beautifully, really. What is it that could come like you said and they are hungry and they want sweets and they bite?

C: What could it be?

H: Yes, you said worms…

C: It could be like a string and maybe this size (HG), 1½ inches. And they are individuals, maybe 3 or 4.

H: So they are like a string, there's like 3 or 4 of them, they bite you, they get hungry, they like sweets, what else can you tell me about this thing? It's like a string…

C: I feel them over a region and it seems like they may be walking or else they just bite.

H: So they could walk and they could bite.

C: Yes. Like that.

H: Could you close your eyes and describe as much as you can about what this thing might be like? In the imagination…does it have color, what's the texture of it? It's like 3 or 4, or it's an inch and a half, it's like a worm.

C: I think it has some kind of head.

H: Very good.

C: And there is a tail. And maybe some little hands.

H: So it's like it has a tail, it has hands, and it has a head, it has a color, anything?

C: The color, I don't know. Maybe pink.

H: And how do you experience theses things, these little things that have a head and could be pink? How do you experience it in your life, having this thing it comes, it goes, what is it like for you to have this? You said you could change your diet…

C: It makes me feel a little bit anxious, and I feel that I must stop and do something.
H: So it makes you feel anxious and like you have to stop and you have to do something. What else?

C: I need to regenerate my body with a new kind of lifestyle.

H: So tell me what regenerate means to you, to regenerate the body?

C: It means to change my habits and change the way that I do things...

H: Okay. Tell me a bit about these worms. You said, you know, in Brazil it's sometimes worms and that this comes and you take a pill, but what are worms?

C: What kind of worms?

H: No, what are worms, tell me about worms, what you know about worms.

C: I think they come and then they clean. But if you grow them inside, it is because you are imbalanced, because you have not been eating well, maybe you don't drink enough water or...

H: No, no. Just tell me about the worms. What are worms? What are the qualities of worms? If you had a child here and they said, what is a worm, because they never saw one, what would you tell them?

C: Oh, what a worm is. I think it's an animal. I don't know. They live in this kind environment that is not scientific. They live in a kind of environment that's no good.

H: That's no good, like...

C: Yes, I say no good, but for them it's good, you know.

H: Good, very good. Tell me about this environment that's no good. Not so much the worm, but what does it mean to be in an environment that's no good.

C: It means that they are there because you don't have a good environment for them to get out of the body. So then they stay there.

H: So just tell me, what is a good environment, not so much for worms, just tell me what's a good and what's a no good environment?

C: I think a good environment is not too much sugar and more exercise.
H: Okay, and a not good environment.

C: A not good environment means like all of this kind of food that we put in the microwave. All processed food. And also this kind of rushing, you know, so then you don't really have time to take care of yourself. Because this is like a cycle.

H: It's like a cycle, this kind of rushing and this cycle, and this waiting the food that goes in the microwave, tell me about this.

C: So this is some kind of routine, but I can't see sometimes another option because I'm feeling forced into this routine. And even if I want to change, and sometimes I have strength, but I'm not strong enough to turn this over. There is some pressure about living without the family and with different people. Even in the church sometimes, it's not...it isn't that fulfillment that I search for. So I started to break these things that I have already learned. Like the knowledge of how to keep the body and the mind okay.

H: You said sometimes you're forced to do that. What is that?

C: Not forced, but you need sacrifice your own needs and give up what you want sometimes to benefit other people. Also, sometimes a situation that you are in forces you to be like this, you know.

H: This I don't get.

C: Like, for example, to cook it takes time. And when I get home from work, my roommates are already sleeping. So I respect my roommates. So then to me it's easier to put the food in the microwave for three minutes instead of making my own food, although I know that to prepare my own food is healthier and could give me more nutrients to live well.

H: So for you, this feeling forced is like in this situation that has to do with that you don't want to bother someone else so it's better to use the microwave so you don't bother them?

C: Yes, in part.

H: What is this? Just explain to me how you see this.

C: I see it like if I share the way that I live with most of the people, they don't understand. Because if I make rice, that's more natural. But it is just harder for to me prepare food from scratch in this kind of environment. I need more people around me who are more comfortable with my ideas. So then I can fit in with what I do. I can try to maintain some balance in everything. But sometimes this balance goes out of my mind.

H: Goes out of your mind, what do you mean?

C: I can't even stop myself, so then I go to sweet things or whatever.

H: So tell me about this kind of environment. You've used this word a few times. Just as if, again, a kid said, what does an environment mean? Not so much your situation because you described it very well, with the food and having people that would understand...

C: So environment is like the house, the fridge, the stove, the pans, the food you get from the market, and the options and the choices that you make to live.

H: And why is this so important to you? Why for you does the environment have to be a good environment? What is this for you?

C: I don't know. I feel that if I am strong, then I can help somebody else. But if I become weak, how can I help any other people? But mostly myself, I need to be strong to do something.

H: And if you're not…what's the opposite? If you're weak, what does that mean?

C: If I'm weak, then I'm going to fail.

H: And what would it mean for you to fail?

C: To fail means not to be focused in my goals.

H: How would you experience it if you were not being focused in your goals and failing? How would you experience that? What would it be like for you if you woke up tomorrow and you were weak and you failed and you could not stay focused on your goals? How would that be for you, in your worst imagination?

C: Like I would need to start over again.

H: For you it would be that you would have to start all over again, what would that be like for you to have to start all over again and build up?

C: I think my main issue relates to meals, to food, this is the main thing that comes to my mind…

H: So tell me everything for you, what is food, this main thing, everything you can tell me…you've told me a lot but just tell me everything you can about this.

C: I would like to be more balanced. To have balance in everything. Like if I need to drink more water, then I'm going to have the water to drink, and I'm not going to skip the water. And if I don't need much sugar, then I won't buy things that contain very much sugar.

H: Very good. Okay, tell me about dreams.

C: My dreams…I have all kinds of dreams. Last night I had a dream with one of my clients. But it was the kind of dream that I didn't want to be there. But…

H: No, tell me about this dream.

C: In the dream my friend, she has some kind of cough, some kind of virus, which was lasting between 3 and 6 months. And the health workers came to her house and they did some exams and they really saw that this was a severe cough. And I told her that I also have a cough and a sore throat. But I don't wish anything bad for them.

H: No, no. This is the imagination, it doesn't matter. Just what happened in the dream?

C: So this is the dream, like I saw it, but I wish it didn't happen. The cough was really annoying to my friend because then her whole family, the kids, like 5 people, had this kind of cough.

H: But, what was it...I don't understand the dream.

C: The dream, I just saw this situation with the family.

H: You saw the situation of the family with this cough. And then what was the feeling?

C: The feeling was that I couldn't do anything.

H: And how did that make you feel?

C: Maybe to wait, to be patient. It was like that.

H: Any other dreams? Any recurring dreams or one that really stands out, even from childhood?

C: They come and they go. But I'm pretty good in the dreams. I remember them and I can act in them.

H: You can act in them, what do you mean?

C: I mean that I can see myself in the dream and then remember everything. And then when I wake up I just reflect about the dream. How does this dream relate to what I am living at this moment? Or what could it show me for the future? Or even some things that it has shown me that were hidden things...

H: Like what? Give me an example.

C: Like one time I had a dream that my pastor was a baby, like a little boy. So that was then a way that I could see him. He is not just a man who screams and is very energetic, on the inside, he is a child.

H: Any other dreams? How about from childhood?

C: From childhood, I was kind of a brat. I was very energetic. We were a family of 6; we were mostly girls and just one brother that came later. But I was punished more than everybody because I always invented something that was not normal, you know.

H: Like what, what was the most unusual thing?

C: Like when I was 6 years old I went with a little boy, under his house porch, to see each other. But my father's office was 2 or 3 blocks away and from his office he saw me. And then he came home and put me inside the home and sent the boy away. So things like that.

H: So you just wanted to look at the body, it was just about looking at the body.

C: Yes, I think so. Sometimes it was not good with my sisters. Actually, just my older sister. Once I was really mad at her. She got an ink pen, but then I took her pen because she wouldn't share it with me. And I pinched her hand with it (HG).

H: You pinched her hand like this (HG)?

C: Yes, and that was very painful for her. But I was always inventing things, extras, you know. I didn't like to be inside much, you know. I preferred to be out in the neighborhood playing and running and stuff like that. Or climbing trees and things like that.

H: Okay, tell me about this cough and this waking in the night and what happens?

C: This cough, it just, it's like, last night I just coughed once and then stopped and then again. It's like something is inside. I relate it somehow with the pulling. And I think the pulling is somehow alive or a living insect that lives and breathes and can stay here (HG to throat), and then they just itch.

H: They itch. And the itch feels like what?

C: It's like they want to get a hole to go inside. And then they make this region feel closed and then this cough (HG).

H: This cough, like this (HG). What is the cough like, the cough itself?

C: My voice feels dirty, not clear, so it's like this region is congested.

H: Like it's…like what? Just use more words here to describe it.

C: Some kind of swell and some kind of flux.

H: But do you cough anything up, does anything come out?

C: No.

H: It's dry or there's something in there?

C: It is dry but there's something behind.

H: It is dry but there's something behind?

C: Yes. Some mucus behind.

H: But you can't get it out.

C: No.

H: And this voice that's dirty but could be clear, what is this?

C: Because I feel something on my ear too. So…

H: What do you feel in your ear?

C: I am very sensitive to the change in the air, too much pressure, or some currents, and so I think it's related to the throat because when the throat is hurting, then I can feel the ear too.

H: So the ear is hurting. Okay, what kind of pain?

C: It just hurts a little. But sometimes I feel fresh air here and I need to put something on it to warm it up and then it goes away.

H: So if you put something warm there, then it feels better?

C: Yes, so when I go to bed at night I pull the blanket up to cover my ear. And then my body warms up and so this goes off.

H: But what do you mean by the voice is dirty and sometimes it's clear?

C: (Clears throat). I need to clear my throat once in awhile.

H: Otherwise what is it?

C: Otherwise I feel some mucus or something stuck.

H: Something is stuck, okay.

C: Yes.

H: And it comes at night mostly?

C: Mostly at night.

H: And it wakes you?

C: Yes.

H: And it comes at these periods, at 2:00 am, at 4:00 am, at 6:00 am, is it like this every night or is it in different patterns?

C: Sometimes it's at 3:00 am, 3:30 am.
H: So this cough it wakes you and then what happens?

C: I just try not to cough very much because of my neighbors and everyone is sleeping in the building, so…but I cough and then I think it has stopped, but then I cough again.

H: Do you think you can give me this cough; can you make this cough now while you're here?

C: (Coughs).

H: Okay, like that. And it comes just once or it comes many at a time? How does it come?

C: No, it comes like a surprise, like you just need to cough and then sometimes you need to cough, cough, cough, and then it comes out.

H: And what comes out?

C: I don't know. Maybe it brings some relief.

H: So you cough, cough, cough, and that's enough? But this wakes you up. But it's better if you drink water, you said?

C: Yes, I feel that if I drink water, its better.

H: Okay, so that's why you're not sleeping, because this cough comes. How long have you had this cough now?

C: Maybe since spring. Like for a month almost.

H: You had it before?

C: Yes, I had it before.

H: The same.

C: Yes, the same thing, and also there is one thing, I sometimes cough so much that I can't contain the cough, and then I might urinate on my bed because there is no way that I can restrain this. So it was much worse before, in the winter. And then I told the doctor about it and he said that if it didn't stop after taking a prescription, that I could have an operation, a surgery, to correct it. But he just mentioned that. He didn't tell me what the problem was exactly.

H: So, now are you taking cough syrup?

C: Now I am taking ginger and honey.

H: Okay, how long have you had this pinching feeling?

C: For more than one month.

H: So this is new too. You had it before?

C: No. This is really new.

H: Okay, tell me about this pain on your foot.

C: This pain is really severe. I have also been to a Chinese medicine practitioner and he said that the pain comes from the kidneys which leads to pain in the legs, but I don't feel pain in my legs.

H: Just tell me about the pain that you felt.

C: It feels like something very heavy is staying there. Or bad circulation maybe. I don't know how to describe it.

H: It feels like something heavy, like what?

C: Yes, like a flat stone or like the muscle is very rigid and then I can't move my fingers very well.

H: Your fingers also?

C: Yes, because the pain is too much.

H: So how does this pain go from your feet to your fingers?

C: I don't know, maybe when I work too hard. I put too much pressure on this part of my body and everything goes through there.

H: So what happens to your fingers?

C: I can't stretch them very well. This pain feels also like congestion, like the pain has to go to everywhere to get out of this point. So then I just feel that I need to walk slowly and put my feet up and relax and that's it, then it goes off.

H: So tell me about the fingers, it's like a point...

C: Yes, usually like if I am driving and if I hold the steering wheel, I feel like my fingers start to go numb, so I can't feel. But it's not as bad as I experienced one or two years ago. Because I used to be a painter and when I had the paint brush in my hands, with the pressure from that, I couldn't feel the tips of my fingers.

H: And when did that start?

C: Maybe two years ago.

H: Okay. You've told me everything about the foot and the fingers the cough the throat?

C: Yes.

H: And why is the losing weight so important to you?

C: Because I feel that I weigh too much, that I need to lose all this stomach I have.

H: And the feeling for you?

C: I want to have more flexibility in my body and more agility to walk and to do work. And also for myself because there are some things that I avoid.

H: Like what?

C: I don't know, like doing things, like I'm getting old.

H: Like what?

C: Like this feeling like I can't do things, like I started to get into some kind of procrastination. And I think that the more I eat, the more I am going to be stuck.

Overview: Client immediately and repeatedly describes discomfort as something "pinching" or "biting" her. Melissa is able to quickly move her to sensation level by providing a lot of encouragement and explaining process and that she wants her to speak from her imagination. Confirms with other complaints: cough, foot pain, finger pain, losing weight.

Chief Complaint: Pinching in side of belly
Vital Expression: pinching (HG) pulling out

Some question homeopath asks about once VE is identified:
Okay, so tell me everything you can about this pinch.
How do you experience these pins on the cloth?
Not this problem you have, because you described really well, just what is this pulling out? As much as you can, use more words...
Like what kind of bites?
What is this attacked, just this one circle? It doesn't have to be this, just whatever comes to mind.
So now just explain to me more about this feeling that comes: it's like sewing, it's like biting, it feels like it could be cancer, that it is an attack...
I'm going to go back. Because you've done beautifully, alright? It's not you, you've done really beautifully, it's just that I'm taking you to a place you've never had to go before. So that's why it will feel quite strange. But actually, you went very quickly, so we'll just go. This feeling, this pulling this biting, I'm going to take you back. Even just close your eyes and just describe with as many different words as you can what the sensation is, how this feels for you. It doesn't have to be exact; whatever comes to mind is really good.
What could this be that's biting like this, just in the imagination, whatever comes?
Could you close your eyes and describe as much as you can about what this thing might be like? In the imagination...
How do you experience it in your life, having this thing it comes, it goes, what is it like for you to have this?

Just tell me about the worms. What are worms? What are the qualities of worms?   If you had a child here and they said, what is a worm, because they never saw one, what would you tell them?

Kingdom Language: animal
This thing comes and maybe it's some kind of alert.
I feel the region is a circle, where they attack me.
Like needles that come in and bite me.
What I feel is that there is something strange in my body. Like I'm growing something different there.
I think they are hungry or they want some sweets, or something.   And if I don't appease them, they come and they give these bites.

Source Language:
It could be like a string and maybe this size (HG), 1½ inches. And they are individuals, maybe 3 or 4.
They may be walking or else they just bite.
I think it has some kind of head.
And there is a tail. And maybe some little hands.
Energy Language:
Maybe pink

Miasm:
It just comes and stays a little bit and then goes off . . . it just comes and goes.
I feel like I need to take better care of my body, to do some cleansing, and to do some limitation. (Malarial)

Remedy: helodrilus caliginosus

Dose: 200c

G. HOMEWORK

Part 1

Give examples for the types of questions you would use at the following points in a case.

1) An opening question
2) At the Fact level within the chief complaint
3) When the patient diverts from the chief complaint
4) At the level of Emotion in order to move to the level of Sensation
5) At the level of Delusion in order to move to the level of Sensation
6) After observing a hand gesture at the level of Sensation, what question would you ask to direct the patient toward sensation language rather than more about the story?
7) A reassurance statement

Part 2

Take a case and observe the hand gestures, body language and any area in the case where there was intense energy. Write about your observations and how they tie into with the totality of the case and its prescription.

Part 3

Make a list of the differences between the Old Method of casetaking and the New Method.

For feedback you can send your homework to Melissa Burch at melissa@innerhealth.us.

About Melissa Burch, CCH

Melissa Burch, CCH, co-founded The Catalyst School of Homeopathy with Christopher Beaver, CCH. She established live phone case supervision and clinics based on the Sensation Method.

She created a unique homeopathic phone referral service with a homeopath team approach. She is president of Inner Health, Inc., which produces numerous online and onsite courses for homeopaths, homeopathic patients and people interested in alternative medicine. She produced the first Radio Series on Homeopathy.

She was the Master Homeopath for the proving of Stoichactis Kenti Sea Anemone. She co-wrote and published the five part "Vital Sensation Manual." Ms. Burch worked with Dr. Nandita Shah at Quiet Healing Center in South India for over a year and half. She graduated from the School of Homeopathy New York, directed by Jo Daly, and the New York School of Homeopathy, directed by Robert Stewart.

About Inner Health, Inc.

Inner Health (IH) provides homeopathic services to the general public and to the homeopathic community. IH is a leader in establishing the highest quality of services in the complementary and alternative medical field through its education, practitioners, workshops and services.

IH's vision is to make homeopathy a household word. Our goal is to identify IH in the consumer's mind as the place to go for the best, natural deep healing on all level— mental, emotional, physical and spiritual; and to create a demand for homeopathy and in particular for Certified IH Homeopaths, through our innovative, educational and creative marketing materials.

Training

IH provides basic and post-graduate training for homeopaths to develop reliable and better results in their practices by following the IH Approach—a systematic way of case taking and analysis based on the Sensation Method—and by implementing the IH System, which includes case management protocols, scripts and information, client business services and marketing.

Homeopaths have the opportunity to train and become Certified IH Homeopaths through workshops, supervision and educational materials. Combined with our own extensive marketing of IH and the IH approach to homeopathy, which results in constant referrals to Certified IH Homeopaths, IH Homeopaths will have a unique and wonderful opportunity to develop themselves as professional homeopaths, heal others, share clinical information with the homeopathic community, be well paid and have excellent systems to guide them to provide the highest care to the client.

www.ingramcontent.com/pod-product-compliance
Lightning Source LLC
Chambersburg PA
CBHW080055280326

41934CB00014B/3327